Cancer Chemotherapy Guidelines and Recommendations for Practice

Second Edition

Editors

Maryanne Fishman, RN, MS

Mary Mrozek-Orlowski, RN, MSN, AOCN®

The Oncology Nursing Society (ONS) would like to thank the original ONS Cancer Chemotherapy Course participants/trainers for their valuable input into this edition, as well as the following original authors:

Jeannie Brant, RN, MS, AOCN®

Aurelie Cormier, RN, CS, MS, AOCN®

Rebecca Hawkins, RN, MSN, ANP, AOCN®

Cindy Johnson, RN

Pamela Kennedy, RN

Maureen O'Rourke, RN, PhD

Mary Beth Riley, RN, MSN, OCN®

Deborah Rust, RN, MSN, CRNP, AOCN®

Charlene Sakuri, RN

Oncology Nursing Press, Inc.
Publisher: Leonard Mafrica, MBA, CAE
Technical Publications Editor: Barbara Sigler, RN, MNEd
Staff Editor: Lisa M. George, BA
Creative Services Assistant: Dany Sjoen

Oncology Nursing Society Education/Cancer Care Issues Team
Linda M. Worrall, RN, MSN, OCN®
Stephanie Jardine, RN, BSN, OCN®
Shelly Slabe, RN, OCN®

Cancer Chemotherapy Guidelines and Recommendations for Practice, Second Edition

Copyright © 1999 by the Oncology Nursing Press, Inc.
Second Printing

Library of Congress Card Catalog Number: 99-62505

ISBN 1-890504-11-4

Publisher's Note

This manual is published by the Oncology Nursing Press, Inc. (ONP). ONP neither represents nor guarantees that the practices described herein will, if followed, ensure safe and effective patient care. The recommendations contained in this manual reflect ONP's judgment regarding the state of general knowledge and practice in the field as of the date of publication. The recommendations may not be appropriate for use in all circumstances. Those who use this manual should make their own determinations regarding specific safe and appropriate patient-care practices, taking into account the personnel, equipment, and practices available at the hospital or other facility at which they are located. The editors and publisher cannot be held responsible for any liability incurred as a consequence from the use or application of any of the contents of these guidelines. Figures and tables are used as examples only. They are not meant to be all-inclusive, nor do they represent endorsement of any particular institution by the Oncology Nursing Society (ONS). Mention of specific products and opinions related to those products do not indicate or imply endorsement by ONS or ONP.

ONS and ONP publications are originally published in English. Permission has been granted by the ONS Board of Directors for foreign translation. (Individual tables and figures that are reprinted or adapted require additional permission from the original source.) However, because translations from English may not always be accurate and precise, ONS and ONP disclaim any responsibility for inaccurate translations. Readers relying on precise information should check the original English version.

Printed in the United States of America

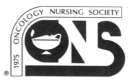

Oncology Nursing Press, Inc.
A subsidiary of the Oncology Nursing Society

Table of Contents

TABLE OF CONTENTS

Introduction

In 1998, the Oncology Nursing Society (ONS) developed a cancer chemotherapy course for nurses. The course content was based on the 1996 *Cancer Chemotherapy Guidelines and Recommendations for Practice*. During the pilot of the course, 50 oncology nurses who are experienced with administering and teaching chemotherapy provided feedback and educational content to both the course and the guidelines. This second edition reflects those changes. Although the practice of administering chemotherapy has not changed drastically over the past few years, newer chemotherapeutic and supportive drugs have changed the way in which we manage patients who receive these agents. Nurses must continue to stay abreast of the latest drugs available.

The second edition of the *Cancer Chemotherapy Guidelines and Recommendations for Practice* reflects the format of the ONS Chemotherapy Course being offered throughout the United States by designated trainers and is utilized as the course handbook. Space is provided throughout the text for nurses to add notes specific to their own practice.

ONS recognizes that nurse practice acts vary from state to state; however, it is the belief of the organization that only registered nurses who receive additional training should administer chemotherapy.

The ONS position regarding the "Preparation of the Professional Registered Nurse Who Administers and Cares for the Individual Receiving Chemotherapy" states the following:

> Specialized preparation of the professional registered nurse can ensure a safe level of care for the individual receiving chemotherapy. This statement defines that position of the ONS regarding the education of the professional registered nurse who administers chemotherapy and cares for these patients.
>
> The ONS *Cancer Chemotherapy Guidelines and Recommendations for Practice* describe basic didactic content and clinical experience necessary for the preparation of the professional registered nurse to care individuals during the treatment continuum and in different settings. Course content includes
>
> - History of cancer chemotherapy
> - Drug development
> - Principles of cancer chemotherapy
> - Chemotherapy preparation, storage, and transport
> - Nursing assessment
> - Chemotherapy administration
> - Safety precautions during chemotherapy administration
> - Disposal, accidental exposure, and spills
> - Institutional considerations
>
> Courses that meet these requirements can prepare professional registered nurses to perform behaviors which can then be evaluated.
>
> The ONS takes the position that the utilization of the content of this publication will provide the information necessary to prepare the professional registered nurse to practice at a safe and competent level.

Every effort has been made to ensure that this manual presents accurate and timely information. Always double-check any information regarding medication dose and administration before administering it to a patient. Nurses who are equipped with knowledge and information are nurses who make a positive impact on the patients for whom they provide care.

The Didactic Component

I. Course Description

The didactic portion of this course is designed to prepare the registered nurse to administer chemotherapy. Relevant topics include

A. Principles of cellular kinetics and pharmacokinetics

B. Chemotherapeutic classifications and specific agents within each classification

C. Safety issues related to drug administration

D. Nursing assessment and management of the patient receiving chemotherapy.

II. Course Objectives

At the completion of the didactic portion of this course, the nurse will be able to

A. Describe historical advances in the field of oncology related to the use of chemotherapy as a treatment modality.

B. Describe the investigational process all drugs undergo for U.S. Food and Drug Administration (FDA) approval.

C. Define the role of the nurse when caring for a patient receiving standard therapy, dose-intensity regimens, and investigational chemotherapy drugs.

D. Identify the importance of the cell cycle and cellular kinetics as they relate to the various chemotherapy classifications.

E. Explain the goals of cancer chemotherapy.

F. Identify methods to measure tumor response to chemotherapy and identify reasons for treatment failure.

G. Describe safety precautions that minimize exposure and untoward effects of chemotherapy to the environment and to the patient, family, healthcare team, and others involved in the handling and disposal of cytotoxic agents.

H. Identify the procedure for administering chemotherapy, including the various routes available and rationale for appropriate selection.

I. Formulate a plan of care for a patient receiving chemotherapy, including data assessment, nursing management, teaching plan, and evaluation criteria.

J. Identify acute, subacute, and chronic toxicities that can occur and describe a care plan to avoid or minimize such side effects.

K. Identify pertinent information in the comprehensive documentation of chemotherapy.

III. Course Content

A. Cancer
1. Definition: Large group of diseases characterized by
   a) Abnormal cell structure
   b) Uncontrolled growth
   c) Ability to spread
   d) Ability to invade normal tissue
2. Grading and differentiation
   a) Grade 1—Well-differentiated
   b) Grade 2—Moderately differentiated
   c) Grade 3—Poorly differentiated
   d) Grade 4—Undifferentiated
3. TNM staging
   a) T = Tumor (local involvement)
   b) N = Node (nodal involvement)
   c) M = Metastasis (distant spread)
4. Treatment modalities
   a) Surgery
   b) Radiation
   c) Chemotherapy
   d) Biotherapy
B. History of cancer chemotherapy (see Table 1)
C. Drug development
1. Preclinical human studies
   a) 10–15-year process
   b) Four steps
      (1) The new agent is discovered either through empirical research (e.g., vincristine [Oncovin®, Eli Lilly and Company, Indianapolis, IN] derived from vinca plant, paclitaxel [Taxol®, Bristol-Myers Squibb Oncology, Princeton, NJ] derived from bark of western yew tree) or rational research of new chemotherapy agents being tested as derivatives that are more effective against cancer or have fewer and less-toxic side effects (e.g., carboplatin [Paraplatin®, Bristol-Myers Squibb Oncology] and idarubicin [Idamycin®, Pharmacia & Upjohn Co., Kalamazoo, MI] analogues of cisplatin [Platinol®, Bristol-Myers Squibb Oncology] and doxorubicin [Adriamycin®, Pharmacia & Upjohn Co.],

Table 1. History of Cancer Chemotherapy

Pre-20th century	1500s: Heavy metals are used systemically to treat cancers; however, they result in limited effectiveness and great toxicity (Burchenal, 1977).
World War I	Sulfur mustard gas is used for chemical warfare; servicemen who are exposed to nitrogen mustard are observed with bone marrow and lymphoid suppression (Gilman, 1963; Gilman & Philips, 1946). Congress passes National Cancer Institute (NCI) Act in 1937.
World War II	Alkylating agents are recognized for their antineoplastic effect (Gilman & Philips, 1946). Thioguanine and mercaptopurine are developed (Guy & Ingram, 1996). 1946: NCI-identified cancer research areas include biology, chemotherapy, epidemiology, and pathology. 1948: Divisions within NCI and external institutions are identified to conduct research (Zubrod, 1984). Folic acid antagonists are found to be effective against childhood acute leukemia (Farber, Diamond, Mercer, Sylvester, & Wolff, 1948).
1950s	Antitumor antibiotics are discovered. National Chemotherapy Program, developed with Congressional funding in 1955, is aimed toward testing and developing new chemotherapy drugs.
1960s–1970s	Development of platinum compounds begins. Multidrug therapy improves remissions without severe toxicity; MOPP (Mustargen®a, Oncovin®b, procarbazine, prednisone), the first combination chemotherapy, is used and found to be curative against Hodgkin's disease (Scofield, Liebman, & Popkin, 1991). Use of chemotherapy with surgery and radiation also is employed as cancer treatment.
1970s	The National Cancer Act of 1971 is created, providing funding for cancer research; director is appointed by and reports to the president of the United States. Doxorubicin phase I trials begin. Use of adjuvant chemotherapy is initiated (Bonadonna et al., 1985; Fisher, Fisher, & Redmond, 1986).
1980s	Community clinical oncology programs (CCOPs) are developed in 1983 to contribute to NCI chemotherapy clinical trials. Multimodal therapies increase in use (Eilber, Morton, Eckardt, Grant, & Weisenburger, 1984; Marcial et al., 1988). Focus turns to symptom management to alleviate dose-limiting toxicities related to neutropenia, nausea and vomiting, and cardiotoxicity. Dexrazoxane (ICRF-187) begins clinical trials as a cardioprotectant (Speyer et al., 1988). New chemotherapeutic agents are available.
1990s	Currently, 35 comprehensive cancer centers, 13 cooperative research groups, and 48 CCOPs are conducting cancer research (NCI, personal communication, January 5, 1999). New classifications of drugs have been developed (e.g., taxanes). Taxol®c (paclitaxel) found to be effective in clinical trials against ovarian and breast cancer (Rowinsky, Onetto, Canetta, & Arbuck, 1992). Biologic-response modifiers and colony-stimulating factors have been developed. U.S. Food and Drug Administration (FDA) approves filgrastim for use in bone marrow transplantation and chemotherapy-induced neutropenia, severe chronic neutropenia, and peripheral blood stem cell transplantation. FDA approves ondansetron for chemotherapy-induced nausea and vomiting; other 5-hydroxytryptamine-3 (5-HT$_3$) receptor antagonists are in clinical trials (Perez, 1995). Dose intensity is becoming a focus, resulting from improved symptom management. FDA approves new analogs (e.g., vinorelbine) (Abeloff, 1995). Additional research on agents continues in combination with biologic response modifiers and potentiators (Yarbro, 1992) and changes in sequencing of agents (Bonadonna, Zambetti, & Valagussa, 1995). Genetic basis of cancers plays important role in cancer risk research (i.e., BRCA1 for breast cancer, renal-cell cancer) (Gnarra, Lerman, Zbar, & Linehan, 1995; Hoskins et al., 1995; Miki et al., 1994). Hormonal therapy makes strides as aromatase inhibitors are approved for breast cancer.

aMerck & Co., Inc., West Point, PA; bEli Lilly and Co., Indianapolis, IN; cBristol-Myers Squibb Oncology, Princeton, NJ

respectively) (Giacalone, 1997).

(2) The agent then is tested *in vitro* in human tumor cell lines from seven different cancers. If the agent is effective, screening is done *in vivo* using mice implanted with cancer cells (Galassi, 1992).

(3) The agent is tested for stability and solubility, and a testing volume is prepared.

(4) The agent is piloted in toxicology studies on animals. The beginning dose for phase I clinical trials in humans is defined (Galassi, 1992).

2. Chemotherapy clinical trials

a) Definition: the study of a new chemotherapy agent or combinations of agents using a scientific experimental design

b) Purpose: to evaluate safety, effectiveness, and toxicities of new chemotherapy drugs and combinations in humans

c) Step-by-step process

(1) Drug is given investigational new drug (IND) approval by the FDA.

(2) The research protocols for the clinical trial are designed in conjunction with the National Cancer Institute (NCI).

(3) Phase I, II, and III clinical trials are partially funded by NCI or private industry (see Table 2).

(4) Clinical drug testing in the United States is completed.

(5) The FDA approves new drug.

(6) Drug can be marketed commercially (Galassi, 1992).

3. The nurse's role in a clinical trial: At many centers, the delivery and monitoring of drugs administered as part of a chemotherapy clinical trial is the role of the research nurse. Therefore, other nurses involved in the care of patients participating in clinical trials may not necessarily be involved in these activities. Communication between nurses involved in the patient's care and the research nurse will help to ensure continuity of care.

a) Phase I

(1) Ensure the patient's eligibility to receive the drug, review preclinical study results for documented side effects and toxicities, and review the investigational drug's action, metabolism, administration

Table 2. Phases of a Clinical Trial for Newly Developed Drugs		
Phase	**Goals**	**Objectives**
I	Initial testing in humans following animal studies Organized as escalating dose trials in which subjects are entered into a series of progressively higher dosage levels until life-threatening, irreversible, or fatal toxicity is experienced	Identify dose-limiting toxicities. Establish maximally tolerated dose, optimal dosage range. Describe pharmacology of agent (e.g., metabolism, distribution, excretion).
II	Testing in selected tumor types ranging from highly chemosensitive to chemoresistant	Determine activity and therapeutic efficacy in a range of tumor types. Validate toxicity and dosage data.
III	Randomized trial comparing new drug with existing therapies in terms of duration and quality of survival; trial may have multiple study arms and involve sample stratification	Determine value of new drug in relation to existing therapies. Generate and publish recommendations for the medical community.
IV	Post-marketing studies	Commercially available Define new uses and dosing schedules. Generate additional information about risks and benefits of new drugs.

Note. From "Clinical Trials: Impact, Evaluation and Implementation Considerations," by C. Engelking, 1993, *Seminars in Oncology Nursing, 8*(2), pp. 148–155; and *The Cancer Chemotherapy Handbook* (4th ed.) (pp. 29–47), by D.S. Fischer, M.T. Knobf, and H.J. Durivage, 1993, St. Louis: Mosby. Adapted with permission.

route, and dosage. The phase I starting dose is usually one-tenth of the maximally tolerated dose in preclinical animal studies (Galassi, 1992).

(2) Serve as an advocate for the patient deciding to enroll in an investigational protocol. This may be a stressful time because the patient may be newly diagnosed with cancer, be experiencing disease progression, or have experienced previous treatment failure (Gross, 1989). No patient is offered a phase I trial if there is a known efficacious treatment that the patient has not received.

(3) Clarify technical explanations of procedures and treatments, and validate the patient's perceptions of the research goal and the risks and benefits involved (Gross, 1989).

(4) Verify that informed consent has been given.

(5) Document pretreatment patient data related to physical and psychosocial exams and understanding of new information (Jenkins & Curt, 1996).

(6) Have emergency equipment available, including monitoring equipment (e.g., monitor/defibrillator, Dinamap® [Critikon, Inc., Tampa, FL]), oxygen, suction, and emergency medications (Galassi, 1992).

(7) Instruct the patient to report changes or symptoms (e.g., shortness of breath, itching, chest pain, chest tightness) during or after drug administration (Galassi, 1992).

(8) Administer the investigational drug; assess, evaluate, and document drug reactions; and use common toxicity criteria to evaluate individual toxicities and identify trends in the study population (see Appendix 1).

(9) Collect frequent timed blood and urine samples for pharmacokinetic monitoring to measure the rate of the drug's metabolism and excretion as appropriate (Jenkins & Curt, 1996).

b) Phase II and III

(1) Review the results of phase I and II studies, including side effects, dose-limiting toxicities, drug metabolism/excretion, and administration route (Giacalone, 1997).

(2) Provide the patient with information about the drug and management of its known side effects.

(3) Assess the patient's understanding of randomization and clarify the meaning of terms (e.g., standard treatment, control group, experimental group) (Giacalone).

(4) Verify that informed consent has been given.

(5) Administer the investigational drug and assess, evaluate, and document drug reactions.

(6) Assess and document symptoms, which may represent therapeutic or toxic side effects of the administered drug.

(7) Follow up with phone calls to assess for delayed or chronic side effects as appropriate (Giacalone). Stress the importance of keeping follow-up appointments.

4. Educational resources

a) Educational resources related to clinical trials can be accessed seven days a week, 24 hours a day, by telephoning 800-4-CANCER. To access information and the fax service at NCI, dial 301-402-5874 (touch-tone dialing). The e-mail address is cancermail@icic.nih.gov.

b) The Physician Data Query (PDQ®) is a computerized informational service that lists available clinical trials and supportive care data for nursing management. Printouts of lists are mailed on request. The Internet address is http://cancernet.nci.nih.gov/pdq.htm.

c) *Taking Part in Clinical Trials: What Cancer Patients Need to Know* (NCI, 1998)

d) NCI videotapes: *Cancer Clinical Trials and You* and *Physician to*

Physician: Perspectives on Clinical Trials.

D. Principles of cancer chemotherapy
  1. Goals of cancer chemotherapy
    a) Cure: Complete response
    b) Control: Extend the length of life when a cure is not realistic
    c) Palliation
      (1) Provision of comfort when cure or control is not possible
      (2) Reduction of tumor burden, thereby relieving associated symptoms, decreasing pain and pressure on nerves and organs, improving vasculature to involved area, relieving organ obstruction, and improving quality of life (Bender, 1998)
    d) Prophylaxis
      (1) Adjuvant
      (2) Neoadjuvant
  2. Tumor cell kinetics and cell life cycle
    a) Cell life cycle: Five-stage reproductive process occurring in both normal and malignant cells (see Figure 1)
      (1) Gap 0 (G_0) resting phase: Cells are temporarily out of cycle and not dividing while all other cellular activities are occurring.
      (2) Gap 1 (G_1) post-mitotic phase: Cells begin an active phase of reproduction. Enzymes necessary for DNA synthesis are produced, and RNA synthesis is occurring.
      (3) Synthesis (S): DNA is produced in preparation for cellular division.
      (4) Gap 2 (G_2): Premitotic or postsynthetic phase: Further protein and RNA synthesis and preparation for mitotic spindles are completed.
      (5) Mitosis (M): Cellular division occurs. The mitotic phase is divided into prophase, metaphase, anaphase, and telephase.
  3. Tumor growth pattern theories (Yarbro, 1992)
    a) Skipper's laws (log-kill model): The first theory is that tumors composed of highly proliferative cells are characterized by exponential growth whereby all cells are dividing, no cells are in a resting phase, and the cell number doubles at a tumor-specific rate, producing an almost constant doubling time. In tumors with

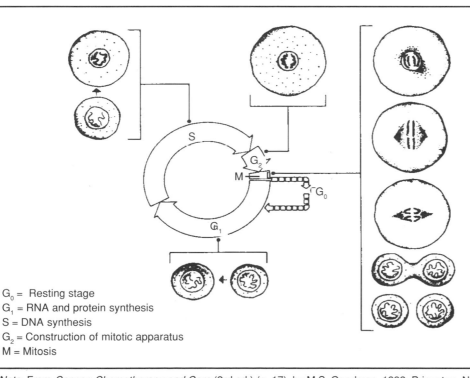

Figure 1. Cell Life Cycle

G_0 = Resting stage
G_1 = RNA and protein synthesis
S = DNA synthesis
G_2 = Construction of mitotic apparatus
M = Mitosis

Note. From *Cancer: Chemotherapy and Care* (3rd ed.) (p. 17), by M.S. Goodman, 1992, Princeton, NJ: Bristol-Myers Squibb Co. Copyright 1992 by Bristol-Myers Squibb Co. Reprinted with permission.

resting cells, this theory only applies to the fraction of cells that are proliferating. The second law is that the percent of cells killed at a given dose is constant in a given tumor (i.e., if a drug kills 90% of the tumor cells, it will kill 90% of the tumor cells regardless of the tumor burden). The log-kill is the logarithm by which the original number of tumor cells must be reduced to equal the remaining cell number.

b) Gompertzian growth: Proliferating tumors behave distinctly differently than nonproliferating tumors. Some cell populations have ceased to proliferate, some have died, and some continue to proliferate. As a result, one population is increasing and one is decreasing. This theory characterizes almost all tumor growth (see Figure 2).

c) Norton-Simon hypothesis: It further elucidates Gompertzian's theory by emphasizing that small tumors have the largest growth fraction because of their high supply of oxygen and nutrients. Conversely, when the total cell number is high, growth fraction is at a minimum because the number of anoxic and necrotic cells has reached a maximum. The purpose of this work was to understand the success and failure of chemotherapy (Norton, 1992).

4. Pharmacology of chemotherapy agents: Chemotherapy is classified according to pharmacologic action of effect on cellular reproduction.

a) Cell-cycle specific drugs exert effect within a specific phase of the cell cycle (see Figure 1).

(1) These drugs have the greatest tumor kill when given in divided doses or as a continuous infusion with a short cycle time.

(2) Classifications include antimetabolites, plant alkaloids, and miscellaneous agents (see Table 3).

b) Cell-cycle nonspecific drugs exert effect in all phases of the cell cycle, including the G_0 resting phase (see Figure 1).

(1) Cell-cycle nonspecific drugs also are effective in treating tumors with fewer dividing cells.

(2) Cell kill is directly proportional to the amount of drug administered.

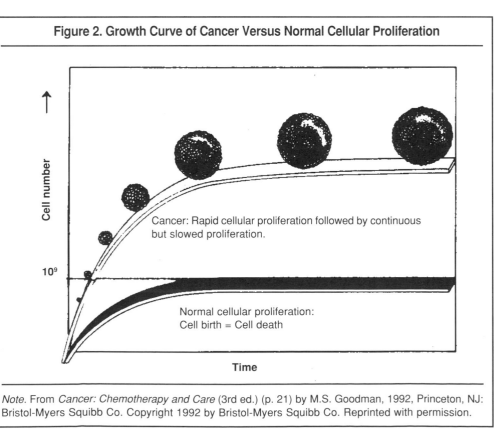

Figure 2. Growth Curve of Cancer Versus Normal Cellular Proliferation

Cancer: Rapid cellular proliferation followed by continuous but slowed proliferation.

10^9

Normal cellular proliferation:
Cell birth = Cell death

Cell number

Time

Note. From *Cancer: Chemotherapy and Care* (3rd ed.) (p. 21) by M.S. Goodman, 1992, Princeton, NJ: Bristol-Myers Squibb Co. Copyright 1992 by Bristol-Myers Squibb Co. Reprinted with permission.

Table 3. Characteristics of Chemotherapy Classification

Classification	Mechanism of Action	Medication Name	Dose*	Indications	Side Effects	Nursing Considerations
Antimetabolites	Act in S phase; inhibit enzyme production for DNA synthesis, leading to strand breaks or premature chain termination	Cytosine arabinoside (cytarabine/AraC)	100 mg/m²/day continuous IV days 1–7 100 mg/m² IV every 12 hours days 1–7	Acute lymphocytic leukemia (ALL), chronic myelocytic leukemia (CML), Hodgkin's and non-Hodgkin's lymphoma	Myelosuppression, nausea, vomiting, anorexia, mucositis, diarrhea, hepatic and renal dysfunction, pruritus, localized pain and/or thrombophlebitis at IV site	· The nurse should make sure the dose ordered is either standard dose or high dose and refer to institutional guidelines. · Also may be ordered intrathecally · Crosses blood-brain barrier · Used mainly with hematologic malignancies
		5-fluorouracil (fluorouracil/5-FU)	500 mg/m² IV days 1–5 450–600 mg/m² weekly 200–400 mg/m² daily as a continuous infusion	Cancers of colon, breast, liver, ovary, pancreas, rectum, stomach	Myelosuppression, nausea, vomiting, diarrhea, mucositis, alopecia, photosensitivity, darkening of veins	· Photosensitivity precautions should take place year-round; encourage sunscreen usage if the patient must be exposed. · Leucovorin often is given concurrently.
		Floxuridine (FUDR)	0.1–0.6 mg/kg/day continuous arterial infusion	Adenocarcinoma of gastrointestinal tract with metastasis to liver, gallbladder, bile ducts	Similar to 5-FU plus abdominal pain, gastritis, enteritis	· Recommendations for dose reductions are for patients with compromised liver function. Monitor patient's hepatic function carefully and adjust dose as per institutional protocol.
		6-mercaptopurine (6-MP/purinethol)	100–200 mg/day PO	Acute leukemia, CML	Myelosuppression, mucositis, nausea, hyperuricemia	· Doses should be reduced by 75% when used concurrently with allopurinol.
		Methotrexate (mexate)	15–30 mg PO or IM days 1–5 every two weeks 12 mg/m² (maximum of 15 mg) intrathecally	Hodgkin's disease, lymphomas and leukemias, central nervous system (CNS) metastasis, cancers of ovary, lung, breast, testes, cervix	Mucositis, nausea, myelosuppression (especially as folic acid antagonist), gastrointestinal ulceration, renal toxicity, photosensitivity	· The nurse should make sure the dose ordered is either standard dose or high dose (high doses are still considered experimental and must be given in conjunction with leucovorin). · Methotrexate does have a few nononcologic indications for its use (e.g., OB/GYN, rheumatoid arthritis).
		6-thioguanine (6-TG/thioguanine)	2 mg/kg/day PO	AML, chronic granulocytic leukemia	Myelosuppression, hyperuricemia, nausea, hepatotoxicity	· No dose reduction is necessary with this drug when used concurrently with allopurinol.
		Fludarabine	25 mg/m² IV for 5 days	Chronic lymphocytic leukemia (CLL)	Bone marrow suppression, nausea, vomiting, diarrhea, rash	· This drug should be given as a 30-minute infusion.
		Capecitabine (Xeloda®)	2,500 mg/m² PO for 14 days, with one week rest	Breast cancer	Diarrhea, hand/foot syndrome, mucositis	· Patient education regarding toxicity reporting/dose reduction is critical.

Cell-Cycle Specific

(Continued on next page)

*All drugs and dosages should be verified with institutional guidelines and/or package inserts prior to administration.

Table 3. Characteristics of Chemotherapy Classification *(Continued)*

Classification	Mechanism of Action	Medication Name	Dose	Indications	Side Effects	Nursing Considerations
Antimetabolites *(cont.)*		Deoxycoformycin (pentostatin)	4 mg/m² IV every other week	Hairy cell leukemia	Fever, nausea, vomiting, and rash; highly toxic at doses more than 10 mg/m² per week; renal failure, confusion, hepatic enzyme elevation	• This drug should be administered with 500 cc–1L of $D_5$1/2NS solution prior to the infusion and 500 cc $D_5$1/2NS solution post infusion.
		Gemcitabine (Gemzar®ᵇ)	1,000 mg/m² IV every week up to 7 weeks	Pancreatic cancer	Myelosuppression especially anemia, nausea, vomiting, fever, flu-like symptoms	• Use with normal saline only • Infuse over 30 minutes; prolongation of infusion time beyond 60 minutes or more than weekly can increase toxicity. • Myelosuppression is a dose-limiting toxicity.
Vinca alkaloids	Act in late G_2 phase, blocking DNA production and in M phase, preventing cell division	Vinorelbine (Navelbine®c)	30 mg/m² IV weekly	Non-small cell lung cancer, breast cancer	Myelosuppression, nausea, vomiting, neurotoxicity, peripheral neuropathy, local tissue necrosis	• Vesicant; should be given IV push over 6–10 minutes through the side port of a free-flowing IV, followed by flushing with 75–125 cc of solution.
	Act in G_1 and S phase by binding to tubulin, inhibiting microtubule formation, also inhibit DNA and RNA formation	Vincristine (Oncovin®ᵇ)	1.4 mg/m² IV weekly (doses should not exceed 2.0 mg)	ALL, Hodgkin's and non-Hodgkin's lymphoma, CML, sarcomas, breast cancer, small cell lung cancer	Peripheral neuropathy, alopecia, constipation—paralytic ileus, jaw pain	• Vesicant; neurotoxicity is cumulative; therefore, it is necessary to do a neuro evaluation prior to each dosing, and dose should be withheld if severe paresthesia, motor weakness, or other abnormalities are present. • Doses should be reduced for significant liver disease. • Stool softeners and/or increased fiber in the diet may help to prevent severe constipation.
		Vinblastine (Velban®ᵇ)	4–18 mg/m² IV weekly	Testicular, squamous cell of head and neck, Hodgkin's lymphoma, Kaposi's sarcoma	Myelosuppression, alopecia, anorexia, jaw pain, peripheral neuropathy, constipation—paralytic ileus	• Vesicant • Generally, neurotoxicity occurs less frequently with vinblastine than with vincristine; however, it can occur with high doses of vinblastine.
Epipodophyllo-toxins	Induce irreversible blockade of cells in pre-mitotic phases of cell cycle, late G_2 and S phase; interfere with topoisomerase II enzyme reaction	Etoposide (VP-16)	50–100 mg/m²/day days 1–5 100 mg/m²/day days 1, 3, 5 Oral dose: Recommendations are generally 2 times the IV dose rounded to the nearest 50 mg.	Cancer of breast and testes, small cell (oat cell) lung cancer, Hodgkin's and non-Hodgkin's lymphoma	Myelosuppression, nausea, vomiting, alopecia, anorexia, orthostatic hypotension, hyperuricemia	• This drug should not be given by rapid IV infusion. It should be infused over 30–60 minutes to avoid hypotension, and blood pressure should be monitored during the infusion. • Prior to use, the drug must be diluted to a final concentration of 0.2–0.4 mg/ml to prevent precipitation.

Cell-Cycle Specific

(Continued on next page)

Table 3. Characteristics of Chemotherapy Classification (Continued)

Classification	Mechanism of Action	Medication Name	Dose	Indications	Side Effects	Nursing Considerations
Epipodophyllo-toxins (cont.)		Teniposide/VM-26 (Vumon®)	165 mg/m² IV twice weekly for 8–9 doses (with cytarabine) 250 mg/m² IV weekly for 4–8 weeks (with vincristine and prednisone)	Childhood ALL	Myelosuppression, hypotension, pulmonary toxicity	· This drug should not be given by rapid IV infusion. It should be infused over 30–60 minutes to avoid hypotension, and blood pressure should be monitored during the infusion. · Allergic reaction · Refer to package inserts for IV preparation and equipment requirements for drug administration.
Taxanes	Stabilize microtubule, thus inhibiting cell division; effective in G₂ and M phase	Paclitaxel (Taxol®)	135–175 mg/m² as a 24-hour infusion every 3–4 weeks 135–175 mg/m² as a 3-hour infusion every 3–4 weeks	Metastatic breast, ovarian, small cell lung cancer	Myelosuppression, alopecia, peripheral neurotoxicity, hypersensitivity reactions, facial flushing, myalgias, fatigue	· The following standard pretreatment regimen must be administered prior to the administration of paclitaxel to help to prevent hypersensitivity reactions including anaphylaxis: Dexamethasone 20 mg PO 12 hours and 6 hours prior to treatment; cimetidine 300 mg IV 30–60 minutes prior to treatment; diphenhydramine 50 mg IV 30–60 minutes prior to treatment · Paclitaxel must be filtered with a 0.2-micron in-line filter. · Paclitaxel should be given in glass bottles or non-PVC bags and through non-PVC tubing. · Paclitaxel is considered a potential vesicant.
		Docetaxel (Taxotere®)	60–100 mg/m² IV every 3 weeks	Breast, non-small cell lung, head and neck, metastatic ovarian cancer	Myelosuppression, hypersensitivity, fluid retention, alopecia, skin and nail changes, mucositis, paresthesia, neurotoxicity	· Patients should be premedicated to reduce the severity of hypersensitivity reactions and fluid retention when receiving docetaxel. The following premedication is necessary prior to dosing: dexamethasone 8 mg PO BID, beginning one day prior and continuing for an additional four days. · Docetaxel must be given through non-PVC tubing. · Refer to additional institutional premedication guidelines.
Camptothecins	Act in S phase; topoisomerase I inhibitor; cause double-strand DNA changes	Topotecan (Hycamtin™)	1.5 mg/m² IV daily for 5 days every 3 weeks	Metastatic ovarian cancer	Myelosuppression, diarrhea, alopecia	· The appropriate volume of reconstituted solution is diluted in either 0.9% sodium chloride IV solution or 5% dextrose IV solution prior to administration.

(Continued on next page)

Table 3. Characteristics of Chemotherapy Classification (Continued)

Classification	Mechanism of Action	Medication Name	Dose	Indications	Side Effects	Nursing Considerations
Camptothecins (cont.)		Irinotecan (Camptosar™g)	125 mg/m² IV weekly for 4 weeks	Metastatic cancer of the colon and rectum	Diarrhea, myelosuppression, alopecia	• This drug can cause both early and late diarrhea, which can be dose limiting. Early diarrhea can occur during or within 24 hours of administration and is generally cholinergic in nature. Atropine is used in many institutional protocols to treat this early diarrhea. Refer to your institutional protocol for dosing and administration of atropine and other antidiarrheals.
Miscellaneous	Inhibit protein synthesis	L-Asparaginase (Elspar®h)	1,000 IU/m²–6,000 IU/m² IM for 10 days. 200 IU/kg/day for 28 days as a single agent	ALL	Nausea, vomiting, hepatotoxicity, fever, hyperglycemia, anaphylaxis	• To prevent hypersensitivity reactions, including anaphylaxis, an intradermal skin test should be given prior to the initial administration of L-asparaginase and repeated if there has been a week or greater time period between doses. • Giving the drug IM greatly reduces the incidence of anaphylaxis.
		Pegaspargase (Oncaspar®e)	2,500 IU/m² IM every 14 days	ALL (for those who have developed hypersensitivity to Elspar)	Hepatotoxicity and coagulopathy	• No need for test dose
	Act in S phase as antimetabolite	Hydroxyurea (Hydrea®i)	20–30 mg/kg PO as a single daily dose 80 mg/kg PO as a single dose every third day (solid tumor doses)	CML, malignant melanoma, squamous cell of head and neck, metastatic ovarian cancer	Myelosuppression, nausea, vomiting, constipation or diarrhea, renal failure, mucositis, hyperuricemia	• Oral agent • The daily dose must be adjusted for blood counts, and the dose should not be changed too frequently because it results in a delay in response.
	May inhibit protein, RNA, and DNA synthesis	Procarbazine (Matulane®a)	100 mg/m² PO daily for 14 days	Hodgkin's disease	Myelosuppression, nausea, vomiting	• Oral agent • Avoid foods high in tyramine because procarbazine exhibits some monoamine oxidase inhibitory activity.
Alkylating agents	Break DNA helix strand, thereby interfering with DNA replication	Busulfan (Myleran®b)	4–8 mg PO total daily dose	CML	Myelosuppression, hyperuricemia, hyperpigmentation, alopecia, gynecomastia, sperm or ovarian suppression	• Monitor blood counts closely, and if the patient's leukocyte count falls below 15,000 u/l, the drug should be discontinued.

Cell-Cycle Specific

Cell-Cycle Nonspecific

(Continued on next page)

Table 3. Characteristics of Chemotherapy Classification (Continued)

Classification	Mechanism of Action	Medication Name	Dose	Indications	Side Effects	Nursing Considerations
Alkylating agents (cont.)		Melphalan (Alkeran®)	6 mg PO daily 2–3 weeks or 16 mg/m² IV every 2 weeks for 4 weeks, then every 4 weeks	Multiple myeloma, ovarian, breast, and testicular cancers, melanoma	Myelosuppression, nausea, vomiting, mucositis, hypersensitivity reactions, tissue necrosis	· Vesicant · Myelosuppression may be delayed and prolonged 4–6 weeks, so monitor blood counts carefully and hold or reduce dose as per institutional protocol.
		Carboplatin (Paraplatin®)	300 mg/m² IV once every 4 weeks with Cytoxan®; 360 mg/m² IV once every 4 weeks as a single agent	Ovarian cancer; cancer of the testes, head and neck, cervix, lung	Thrombocytopenia, neutropenia (myelosuppression more pronounced with renal impairment), nausea, vomiting, renal/hepatic toxicity uncommon	· Carboplatin exhibits much less renal toxicity than cisplatin, so there is no need for rigorous hydration. · Bone marrow suppression is the dose-limiting toxicity, especially thrombocytopenia. Monitor blood counts closely and dose reduce as per protocol.
		Cisplatin (CDDP, Platinol®)	75–100 mg/m² IV once every 3–4 weeks when used with Cytoxan; 100 mg/m² IV once every 3–4 weeks as a single agent	Cancers of cervix, ovary, endometrium, bladder, prostate, esophagus, kidney, testes; non-small cell of lung; squamous cell carcinoma of head and neck; osteogenic sarcomas; bone marrow transplant	Severe nephrotoxicity, nausea, vomiting, myelosuppression, ototoxicity, hyperuricemia	· Vesicant potential if > 20 cc of 0.5 mg/ml extravasated. If less, drug is an irritant. · It is recommended to hold the drug if the patient's serum creatinine is > 1.5 mg/dl, as irreversible renal tubular damage may occur. · Rigorous hydration is necessary to prevent nephrotoxicity. · Cisplatin can cause ototoxicity; therefore, a baseline audiogram should be done.
		Cyclophosphamide (Cytoxan®)	40–50 mg/kg IV given in divided doses over 2–5 days 10–15 mg/kg IV every 7–10 days 3–5 mg/kg IV twice weekly Oral doses: 400 mg/m² PO days 1–5 every 3–4 weeks or 60–120 mg/m² PO daily	Cancers of breast, lung, prostate, ovary, head and neck; multiple myeloma; leukemias; lymphomas; Wilms' tumor	Hemorrhagic cystitis, vomiting, myelosuppression, nausea, alopecia, syndrome of inappropriate antidiuretic hormone	· Give the dose, whether it be IV or oral, in the morning, adequately hydrate the patient, and if it is oral, have the patient drink plenty of fluids. · Have the patient empty bladder frequently to prevent hemorrhagic cystitis.
		Ifosfamide (Ifex®)	1.2 g/m² IV days 1–5 every 3–4 weeks Mesna 240 mg/m² IV at 0, 4, 8 hours (recommended dosing schedule with ifosfamide).	Cancers of lung, testes, and marrow; non-Hodgkin's lymphoma; sarcomas	Hemorrhagic cystitis, nausea, alopecia, vomiting, myelosuppression	· Administer the drug over 30 minutes or more. · To prevent hemorrhagic cystitis, always give with mesna. Mesna may be given as a bolus dose, continuous infusion, or mixed in the bag with the ifosfamide. The mesna dose should be 20% of the ifosfamide dose (based on weight).

Cell-Cycle Nonspecific

(Continued on next page)

Table 3. Characteristics of Chemotherapy Classification (Continued)

Classification	Mechanism of Action	Medication Name	Dose	Indications	Side Effects	Nursing Considerations
Alkylating agents *(cont.)*		Mechlorethamine hydrochloride (nitrogen mustard)	6 mg/m² IV days 1 and 8 every 4 weeks (MOPP for Hodgkin's disease)	Hodgkin's disease, CLL, CML	Severe nausea, vomiting, alopecia, myelosuppression, pain or phlebitis at IV site, chills, fever	· Vesicant · Administer the drug over several minutes through the side arm of a freeflowing IV, taking care not to extravasate! · Flush with 125–150 cc of normal saline. · If extravasation should occur, sodium thiosulfate is the antidote. · Mechlorethamine should be used as soon after preparation as possible (15–30 minutes) as it is extremely unstable. · Mechlorethamine must not be mixed with any other drug.
		Thiotepa	0.3–0.4 mg/kg IV (doses given at 1–4-week intervals) 0.6–0.8 mg/kg intracavitary administration	Cancers of bladder, breast, ovary, Hodgkin's disease, lymphomas	Myelosuppression, ovarian or sperm suppression, nausea, vomiting, pain at infusion site, rash, fever	· The drug is primarily excreted in the urine; renal function should be carefully monitored.
		Chlorambucil (Leukeran®c)	3–4 mg/m² PO daily until a response or cytopenias occur, then maintain if necessary with 1–2 mg/m² PO daily.	CLL, Hodgkin's disease	Myelosuppression, ovarian or sperm suppression, nausea, vomiting	· Increased in toxicity may arise if the patient was on barbiturates previously.
Antitumor antibiotics	Bind with DNA, thereby inhibiting DNA, RNA synthesis	Bleomycin (Blenoxane®)	10–20 units/m² IV, IM, or SQ weekly or twice weekly	Pleural effusion in carcinoma of lung; squamous cell of head and neck; cancer of cervix, vulva, penis, testes; Hodgkin's disease; lymphoma	Hypersensitivity or anaphylactic reaction (rare), hyperpigmentation, alopecia, photosensitivity, renal/hepatotoxicity, pulmonary fibrosis, fever, chills	· There is an increased incidence of anaphylaxis with lymphoma patients; therefore, an IM or SQ test dose of 1–2 units is recommended prior to the first dose of bleomycin. · The cumulative lifetime dose should not exceed 400 units because of the dose-related incidence of pulmonary fibrosis.
		Dactinomycin (actinomycin D)	500 mcg (0.5 mg) IV daily for a maximum of 5 days	Ewing's sarcoma, Wilms' tumor, testicular cancer, choriocarcinoma	Myelosuppression, nausea, vomiting, alopecia, mucositis, diarrhea, ovarian or sperm suppression, radiation recall (hyperpigmentation of previously radiated areas)	· Vesicant · This drug may be ordered in mcg, so carefully check the dose. · Dactinomycin may cause "radiation recall" to previously irradiated skin or even irritated skin.

Cell-Cycle Nonspecific

(Continued on next page)

Table 3. Characteristics of Chemotherapy Classification *(Continued)*

Classification	Mechanism of Action	Medication Name	Dose	Indications	Side Effects	Nursing Considerations
Antitumor antibiotics *(cont.)*		Daunorubicin (daunomycin)	45mg/m² IV push days 1, 2, 3 first course for patients < 60 years old; 30 mg IV push days 1, 2, 3 first course for patients > 60 years old	ALL in children, acute nonlymphocytic leukemia	Myelosuppression, nausea, vomiting, alopecia, cardiotoxicity, hyperuricemia, radiation recall, ovarian or sperm suppression, drug excreted as a red color in urine	• Vesicant • This drug may cause the patient's urine to turn a red color. • The patient's cardiac function (ejection fraction) should be tested via MUGA scan prior to starting therapy with this agent. • The dose generally is less if the patient is more than 60 years of age (example: > 60 years, 30 mg/m² versus < 60 years, 45 mg/m²).
		Doxorubicin (Adriamycin®)	60–75 mg/m² IV every 3 weeks as a single agent 40–60 mg/m² IV every 21–28 days in combination with other drugs	Cancer of breast, ovary, prostate, stomach, thyroid; small cell lung, liver; squamous cell of head and neck, multiple myeloma, Hodgkin's disease, lymphomas, ALL, AML	Myelosuppression, nausea, vomiting, alopecia, mucositis, dose-limiting cardiotoxicity, radiation recall, arrhythmias, hyperuricemia, photosensitivity, drug excreted as a red color in urine	• Vesicant • A flare reaction can occur. • The patient's cardiac function (ejection fraction) should be tested via MUGA scan prior to starting therapy with this agent. • It is recommended not to exceed a lifetime cumulative dose of 550 mg/m² (450 mg/m² if the patient has had prior chest radiation or concomitant cyclophosphamide). • This drug may cause the patient's urine to turn a red color. • Patients who have received a cumulative dose of 300 mg/m² and are continuing doxorubicin treatment should have dexrazoxane initiated.
		Idarubicin (Idamycin®)	12 mg/m² IV daily for 3 days (induction)	Acute nonlymphocytic leukemia	Myelosuppression, nausea, vomiting, alopecia, vein itching, cardiomyopathy, radiation recall	• Vesicant • Cardiac toxicity is less than that with daunorubicin. Cumulative doses > 150 mg have been associated with decreased ejection fractions. • Local reactions such as hives at the injection site may occur.
		Mitomycin-C (Mitomycin®)	20 mg/m² IV once every 6–8 weeks	Cancers of pancreas, stomach, colon, breast, lung, bladder, esophagus, head and neck, multiple myeloma	Myelosuppression, alopecia, mucositis, renal and pulmonary toxicity, fatigue	• Vesicant • Nadir is 4–8 weeks. • Acute shortness of breath and bronchospasm can occur very suddenly when this drug is given simultaneously or concurrently with a vinca alkaloid.

Cell-Cycle Nonspecific

(Continued on next page)

Table 3. Characteristics of Chemotherapy Classification *(Continued)*

Classification	Mechanism of Action	Medication Name	Dose	Indications	Side Effects	Nursing Considerations
Antitumor antibiotics *(cont.)*		Mitoxantrone (Novantrone®k)	12–14 mg/m² every 21 days	Breast cancer, lymphomas, acute nonlymphocytic leukemia	Myelosuppression, arrhythmias if treated previously with doxorubicin, drug excreted as a blue-green color in urine, can also cause blue discoloration of the sclera	· Vesicant · Cardiac toxicity is less than with doxorubicin, but any prior anthracycline use, chest irradiation, or cardiac disease can increase the patient's risk.
		Plicamycin (Mithracin®k)	25–30 mcg/kg IV for 8–10 days For hypercalcemia: 25 mcg/kg for 3–4 days	Testicular cancer	Myelosuppression, nausea, vomiting, diarrhea, mucositis, hypokalemia, hypocalcemia, hypophosphatemia, facial flushing, phlebitis, renal/ hepatic toxicity	· The most important toxicity associated with the use of this drug is a bleeding syndrome, which usually begins with an episode of epistaxis. · Monitor blood counts, especially platelets. · The drug should be administered over 30 minutes to reduce gastrointestinal toxicity.
Hormonal therapy	Interferes with hormone receptors and proteins in all phases of cell cycle	Glucocorticoids Prednisone, hydrocortisone, Solu-Medrol®g, dexamethasone i (Decadron®l)	Refer to specific protocols for doses of the agents listed, as they will vary depending on specific reasons for use.	Cancer of breast with hypercalcemia, Hodgkin's disease, multiple myeloma, lymphoma, leukemias, cerebral/spinal cord primary and metastatic tumors	Fluid and sodium retention, hyperglycemia, gastrointestinal irritation, masks infection, hypokalemia; long-term therapy, hypertension, osteoporosis, cushingoid appearance, cataracts or glaucoma, mood alteration, perineal burning with rapid infusion	· Stress the importance of schedule maintenance with steroids, especially if it is part of the treatment regimen.
		Estrogens Chlorotrianisene (TACE), diethylstilbestrol (DES), Estratab®g, stradiol	TACE: 12–25 mg PO daily DES: 1–3 mg PO daily, can later reduce to 1 mg PO daily Estratab: 1.25–2.5 mg PO 3 times daily for at least 3 months	Prostate cancer, estrogen receptor-positive breast tumors, postmenopausal advanced breast cancer	Gynecomastia, breast tenderness, fluid and sodium retention, nausea, vomiting, thrombophlebitis, libido changes, voice deepening	· Women with an intact uterus should be monitored for signs of endometrial cancer.
		Anti-Estrogens Tamoxifen (Nolvadex®d)	10 mg tab PO twice daily	Estrogen receptor-positive, postmenopausal breast cancer	Menstrual irregularities, vaginal bleeding or discharge, hot flashes, nausea, vomiting, edema, hypercalcemia	· Adverse reactions are relatively mild and rarely severe enough to require discontinuation of treatment.

(Continued on next page)

Cell-Cycle Nonspecific

Table 3. Characteristics of Chemotherapy Classification (Continued)

Classification	Mechanism of Action	Medication Name	Dose	Indications	Side Effects	Nursing Considerations
Hormonal therapy (cont.)		Progestins Medroxyprogesterone acetate (Depo-Provera®m), megestrol acetate (Megace®g)	Medroxyprogesterone acetate: 400–1,000 mg IM per week initially Megestrol acetate: 40 mg 4 times a day; for endometrial cancer: 40–320 mg/day in divided doses	Breast cancer, metastatic renal cell carcinoma	Fluid retention, headache, nausea, vomiting, vaginal bleeding or spotting, thrombophlebitis	· At least two months of continuous treatment is considered an adequate period for determining the efficacy of megestrol acetate.
		Leuprolide (Lupron®m)	Refer to specific protocols for doses of the agents listed, as they will vary depending on specific reasons for use.	Prostate cancer	Gynecomastia, hot flashes, nausea, vomiting, headache, bone pain	· It is important to maintain the prescribed dose and schedule of drug. · Go over all side effects with the patient prior to administration of drug and inform the patient that worsening of symptoms may occur in the first few weeks of therapy.
Nitrosoureas	Break DNA helix, interfering with DNA replication; cross blood-brain barrier	Carmustine (BCNU)	75–100 mg/m² IV every day for 2 days or 150–200 mg/m² IV as a single dose	Hodgkin's disease, non-Hodgkin's lymphoma, CNS tumors, multiple myeloma, malignant melanoma, bone marrow transplant	Nausea, vomiting, myelosuppression, renal/hepatic toxicity, pulmonary fibrosis, ovarian or sperm suppression	· The nadir occurs between 4–6 weeks. · Because of delayed toxicity, successive treatments usually are given no more frequently than every 6–8 weeks. · Rapid infusion may cause burning along the vein and flushing of the skin. · Long-term therapy can result in pulmonary fibrosis, which may present as an insidious cough and dyspnea or sudden respiratory failure. · Crosses blood-brain barrier.
		Lomustine (CCNU)	100–130 mg/m² PO as a single oral dose every 6 weeks	Pancreatic, liver, gastric, colorectal cancer; CNS tumors, multiple myeloma, Hodgkin's disease	Myelosuppression (severe), nausea, vomiting, alopecia, renal/hepatic toxicity, mucositis	· The dose should not be repeated more often than every six weeks due to delayed myelosuppression. · Crosses blood-brain barrier.
		Streptozocin (Zanosar®g)	1.0–1.5 g/m² every week **or** 500 mg/m² every day for 5 days **Do not exceed 1.5 g/m²**	Islet cell pancreatic carcinoma (metastatic)	Renal toxicity, myelosuppression, nausea, vomiting, hyperglycemia, proteinuria	· Nephrotoxicity may be dose limiting. · This drug may alter glucose metabolism in some patients. · Rapid infusion may cause burning along the vein.

Cell-Cycle Nonspecific

a Hoffmann-La Roche Inc., Nutley, NJ; b Eli Lilly and Co., Indianapolis, IN; c Glaxo Wellcome Oncology/HIV, Research Triangle Park, NC; d Bristol-Myers Squibb Oncology, Princeton, NJ; e Rhône-Poulenc Rorer Pharmaceuticals, Inc., Collegeville, PA; f SmithKline Beecham Pharmaceuticals, Philadelphia, PA; g Pharmacia & Upjohn Co., Kalamazoo, MI; h Merck & Co., West Point, PA; i Immunex Corp., Seattle, WA; j Adria Laboratories, Dublin, OH; k Miles Inc., West Haven, CT; l Zeneca Pharmaceuticals, Wilmington, DE; m TAP Pharmaceuticals, Deerfield, IL

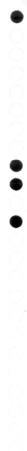

_____

_____

_____

_____

_____

_____

_____

_____

_____

_____

_____

_____

_____

_____

_____

_____

_____

_____

_____

_____

(3) Classifications include alkylating agents, antitumor antibiotics, hormonal therapy, and nitrosourea agents (see Table 3).

5. Factors affecting response

a) Tumor burden: The inverse relationship between the number of tumor cells and chemotherapeutic response implies that the smaller the tumor, the higher the rate of cure.

b) Combination versus single-agent therapy

(1) Combination chemotherapy is able to increase the proportion of cells killed at any one time.

(2) Combination chemotherapy reduces the possibility of drug resistance by using drugs that have different mechanisms of action (Bertino & O'Keefe, 1992).

(3) Combination chemotherapy uses the principle of drug synergy to maximize the effects of another drug. Synergy is affected by the proliferative rate of tumor growth as well as by whether the drugs are administered sequentially or simultaneously (e.g., leucovorin can potentiate fluorouracil's cytotoxicity) (Finley, 1992).

(4) Agents selected for use in combination chemotherapy have a proven efficacy as single agents and have minimally overlapping organ toxicity.

c) Hormone receptor status

d) Administration schedule

(1) Bolus therapy

(2) Infusional therapy (parenteral therapy for more than 24 hours): As the practice of infusional therapy continues to evolve, clinical trials strive to improve the therapeutic index and decrease toxicity by testing various infusional applications. Examples of new multiagent infusional patterns include the following.

(a) Simultaneous infusion of multiple agents (e.g., cisplatin, leucovorin, calcium, 5-fluorouracil)

(b) Simultaneous administra-

tion of admixtures of pharmaceutically compatible antineoplastic agents

(c) Sequential alternating infusions of incompatible agents (e.g., cyclophosphamide, methotrexate, and fluorouracil [CMF] or cytoxan, doxorubicin, fluorouracil [CAF]) (Anderson & Lokich, 1994)

(d) Combined modality therapy: use of chemotherapy and radiation or surgery as primary, neoadjuvant, simultaneous, or adjuvant treatment

e) Dose category

(1) High dose entails administering sufficient drug to potentially eradicate tumor but to cause sufficiently severe side effects to warrant supportive therapy (e.g., granulocyte-colony stimulating factor [G-CSF] as supportive therapy for neutropenia) (see Table 4).

(2) Dose intensification entails using higher than standard dose (10–200 times standard dose) (Petros & Peters, 1993). Dose intensification may be administered as

(a) Single high dose

(b) Divided fractional dose over two or more days (may enhance cell kill)

(c) Long-term infusion: Dose is administered as a continuous infusion for one to several days (may minimize side effects).

f) Drug resistance: phenomenon by which a cancer cell becomes resistant to antineoplastic agent(s), which ultimately interferes with the ability to fight the tumor

(1) Intrinsic or permanent resistance occurs when cells become resistant to antineoplastic agents at the time of malignant cell transformation (prior to exposure to antineoplastic agents).

(2) Acquired resistance occurs when malignant cells become resistant to antineoplastic agents after exposure to them. Malignant cell lines may be

Table 4. Common Agents Used in Dose-Intensive/High-Dose Chemotherapy and Associated Toxicities

Drug	Toxicity
Doxorubicin	1. Cardiotoxicity leading to degenerative cardiomyopathy over time (Lindower & Skorton, 1992) Standard dose: 60–75 mg/m^2 Current lifetime dose: 450–550 mg/m^2 Current protocol dose ranges: 430–650 mg/m^2 (lifetime) When given over 96 hours in a dilute solution or at low weekly doses, cardiotoxicity appears to decrease. Prior radiation therapy to the chest or prior anthracycline therapy may predispose patient to or enhance cardiotoxicity. 2. Severe mucositis 3. Acute myelosuppression; late onset in children, even at low cumulative doses
Cyclophosphamide	1. Standard dose: 400–1,600 mg/m^2 IV; high dose: up to 200 mg/kg 2. High dose: Cardiotoxicity, acute cardiomyopathy (Gardner et al., 1993) Diminished QRS complex on ECG Pulmonary congestion and pleural effusions Cardiomegaly Prior radiation therapy to the chest or prior anthracycline therapy may predispose patient to or enhance cardiotoxicity Ejection fraction of > 50% not predictive of reduced risk for cardiotoxicity 3. Hemorrhagic cystitis (occasionally chronic, severe) 4. Acute myelosuppression 5. Acral erythema and sloughing of skin on palms of hands and soles of feet 6. Diffuse hyperpigmentation 7. Gonadal dysfunction Delayed pubertal development Diminished testicular volume in adult males
Cisplatin	1. Standard dose: 15–120 mg/m^2; high dose: 160–200 mg/m^2 2. Renal and hepatic toxicity 3. Eighth cranial nerve damage and ototoxicity 4. Myelosuppression 5. Peripheral neuropathy 6. Intense nausea and vomiting
Carboplatin (Calvert, Newell, & Gore, 1992; Ozols, Ostchega, Curt, & Young, 1987)	1. Standard dose: 400–500 mg/m^2; high dose: 800–1,600 mg/m^2 2. Myelosuppression (dose-limiting); pronounced thrombocytopenia 3. Severe nausea and vomiting 4. Hepatotoxicity 5. Auditory toxicity 6. Mild renal toxicity
Cytosine arabinoside	1. Standard dose: 100–200 mg/m^2; high dose: 2–3 g/m^2 2. Acute neurotoxicity: cerebellar toxicity Those over 50 at highest risk for minimal recovery from symptoms. Assess prior to each dose for ataxia, nystagmus, and slurred speech; hold dose if any indication of symptomatology (over baseline assessment). 3. Acral erythema and possible sloughing of skin on palms of hands and soles of feet 4. Conjunctivitis Steroid eye drops may prevent or alleviate 5. Intense diarrhea, up to 2–3 liters/24 hours
Busulfan	1. Standard dose: 1–4 mg/m^2; high dose: 16 mg/kg 2. Myelosuppression 3. Severe nausea and vomiting 4. Severe mucositis 5. Pneumonitis, pulmonary fibrosis; "busulfan lung" 6. Hepatic dysfunction leading to veno-occlusive disease 7. Diffuse hyperpigmentation; rare: development of bullae 8. Chronic alopecia (Baker et al., 1991)

(Continued on next page)

Table 4. Common Agents Used in Dose-Intensive/High-Dose Chemotherapy and Associated Toxicities *(Continued)*

Drug	Toxicity
Etoposide	1. Standard dose: 60 mg/m²; high dose: 60 mg/kg or 80–250 mg/m² 2. Severe mucositis 3. Acral erythema and sloughing of skin on palms of hands and soles of feet 4. Myelosuppression 5. Severe blood pressure fluctuations 6. Fever and chills during infusion
Methotrexate	1. Standard dose: 10–500 mg/m²; high dose: 500 mg/m² and greater 2. Photosensitivity 3. Diffuse hyperpigmentation 4. Neurotoxicity: seizures, aphasia, cerebellar toxicity (rare; see cytosine arabinoside) 5. Severe diarrhea 6. Renal toxicity 7. Hepatotoxicity and coagulopathies (Skeel, 1991) 8. Thrombocytopenia 9. Pulmonary toxicities
Melphalan	1. Standard dose: 6–8 mg/m²; high dose: 80–140 mg/m² 2. Severe mucositis 3. Diarrhea 4. Severe nausea, especially in combination with another emetogenic drug 5. Renal toxicity 6. Profound myelosuppression 7. Severe liver toxicity
Carmustine	1. Standard dose: 200–240 mg/m²; high dose 600–1,200 mg/m² 2. Hepatic dysfunction leading to veno-occlusive disease 3. Central nervous system changes, including diffuse encephalopathy 4. Mild alopecia
5-Fluorouracil	1. Standard dose: 7–15 mg/kg for five days; high dose: 255–300 mg/m² continuous infusion weekly 2. Cardiotoxicity mimicking acute myocardial infarction, angina, cardiogenic shock 3. Photosensitivity and hyperpigmentation 4. Severe diarrhea 5. Cerebellar toxicity

resistant to single antineoplastic agents and to other structurally dissimilar antineoplastic agents (e.g., pleiotropic resistance, multidrug resistance). Strategies have been developed to overcome some of the biochemical variables that influence resistance. As a result, the terms relative or temporary resistance also may be used (Moscow & Cowan, 1988; Tortorice, 1997). The following resistance mechanisms are commonly described, although others exist.

(a) Classical multidrug resistance (MDR-1) is cross resistance to unexposed drugs of a different drug classification after exposure to one antineoplastic drug. P-glycoprotein acts to eject antineoplastic agents from the cell.

(b) Atypical multidrug resistance, topoisomerases: Topoisomerases (enzymes vital for cell division) are inhibited or altered by several antineoplastic agents, causing resistance to these drugs.

(c) Glutathione (GSH) and glutathione S-transferase (GST) isoenzymes: Isoenzymes are important in DNA synthesis and repair. GSH and GST may contribute to altering the activation of some antineoplastic drugs by neutralizing cell toxins.

g) Factors that may lessen chemotherapy morbidity and mortality
   (1) Supportive therapies (e.g., prophylactic antibiotics, antiemetics, intensive blood products support, nutritional support)
   (2) G-CSF and granulocyte-macrophage CSF (GM-CSF)
      (a) Shorten the period of severe myelosuppression
      (b) Decrease the risk and incidence of neutropenic sepsis and shorten hospital stays
      (c) Are successfully used with standard-dose and high-dose chemotherapy (Crawford et al., 1991; Gabrilove et al., 1988)
      (d) Recombinant human erythropoietin alfa
      (e) Thrombopoietic growth factor, IL-11
6. Measuring tumor response
   a) Complete response: absence of all signs and symptoms of cancer for at least one month using objective criteria (e.g., quantitative bidimensional tumor measurement)
   b) Partial response: at least a 50% reduction of measurable tumor mass for one month without development of new tumors
   c) Stable disease: less than a 50% reduction or less than a 25% increase of cancer growth
   d) Progression: 25% or greater growth or development of new tumors
   e) Subjective response: The patient's perception that he or she feels better, is gaining weight, and is more active despite no demonstration of improvement in objective parameters
   f) Measurement criteria
      (1) Performance scale: Karnofsky Performance Status Scale (see Table 5), the American Joint Committee on Cancer, and the Zubrod Scale
      (2) Tumor assessment: surgical examination, physical examination, imaging studies (e.g.,

Table 5. Performance Status Scales

Zubrod Rating	General Category	Karnofsky Percent	Specific Performance
0	Able to carry on normal activity; no special care needed	100	Normal; no complaints; no evidence of disease
		90	Able to carry on normal activity; minor signs or symptoms of disease
		80	Normal activity with effort; some signs or symptoms of disease
1	Unable to work; able to live at home and to care for most personal needs; a varying amount of assistance needed	70	Care for self; unable to carry on normal activity or do active work
2		60	Occasional assistance; able to care for most of needs
		50	Considerable assistance and frequent medical care
3	Unable to care for self; equivalent of institutional or hospital care; disease may be progressing rapidly	40	Disabled; special care and assistance
		30	Severely disabled; hospitalization; death not imminent
		20	Very sick; hospitalization necessary
4	Completely disabled	10	Moribund; fatal processes progressing rapidly
5		0	Dead

Note. From "Principles of Cancer Research," by L. Meili, in S. Otto (Ed.), *Oncology Nursing* (p. 354) 1991, St. Louis: Mosby-Year Book. Copyright 1991 by Mosby-Year Book. Adapted with permission.

computerized tomography [CT] scan, x-rays, magnetic resonance imaging [MRI], nuclear medicine scans), and serum tumor markers (e.g., carcinoembryonic antigen [CEA], prostate-specific antigen [PSA], Ca 27.29)

(3) Survival data

7. Cancer chemotherapeutic agents (see Table 3)

E. Pretreatment phase

1. Nursing assessment

a) Patient history

(1) Recent treatment, including surgery, prior chemotherapy (including dose, route, usage in disease, and, if appropriate, investigational protocol), radiation, and biologic or hormonal therapy

(2) Medical and surgical history as appropriate, including allergies

(3) Psychosocial status of the patient, significant other, and family, including cultural issues

(4) Review of systems to assess for any side effects from previous treatments or disease progression

(5) Assessment of physical performance status using a quantitative scale (e.g., Karnofsky)

(6) Obtain height and weight.

(7) Review of previous and current laboratory data, including

(a) Complete blood count (CBC) with differential

(b) Liver and renal function tests

(c) Electrolytes; blood, urea, nitrogen (BUN); serum creatinine

(8) Review of tumor type, stage, and grade

b) Patient and family education

(1) Assess primary language and level of understanding, culture, ability to read, readiness to learn, anxiety, and other potential barriers to learning, as well as desired level of decision making and participation in care (Grahan & Johnson, 1990).

(2) Identify educational materials, considering learning style and

preference, primary language, reading level, and cultural background.

(3) Address various educational topics.

(a) Treatment plan or protocol

(b) Treatment goals

(c) Drug names

(d) Side effects and rationale for frequency of laboratory tests

(e) Strategies to manage side effects at home

(f) When to call nurse/physician

(4) Provide names and numbers (e.g., clinic, home-infusion firm, physician) for the patient and family to call (Wickham, Purl, & Welker, 1992).

c) Treatment plan review

(1) Compare written orders to formal drug protocol or reference source (e.g., chemotherapy text) and identify the therapy prescription and administration route. Recalculate the dose and check against the order.

(2) Review of vesicant/irritant potential of drugs

(3) Determination of drug dose

(a) Calculate according to milligrams per kilogram (mg/kg) of body weight or milligrams per meter squared (mg/m^2) by body surface area (BSA) for both adults and children. (BSA is more accurate and widely used for adults.)

(b) To measure BSA, use the following mathematical calculation:

$$\sqrt{\dfrac{\text{height x weight}}{3,600}}$$

or use a BSA calculator or nomogram scale (see Figure 3).

(c) Multiply the BSA by the amount of drug ordered.

(d) Exceptions: Standard recommended doses may require modification in certain situations.

i) For patients who are obese, ideal body weight

Figure 3. Estimation of Surface Area From Height and Weight[a]

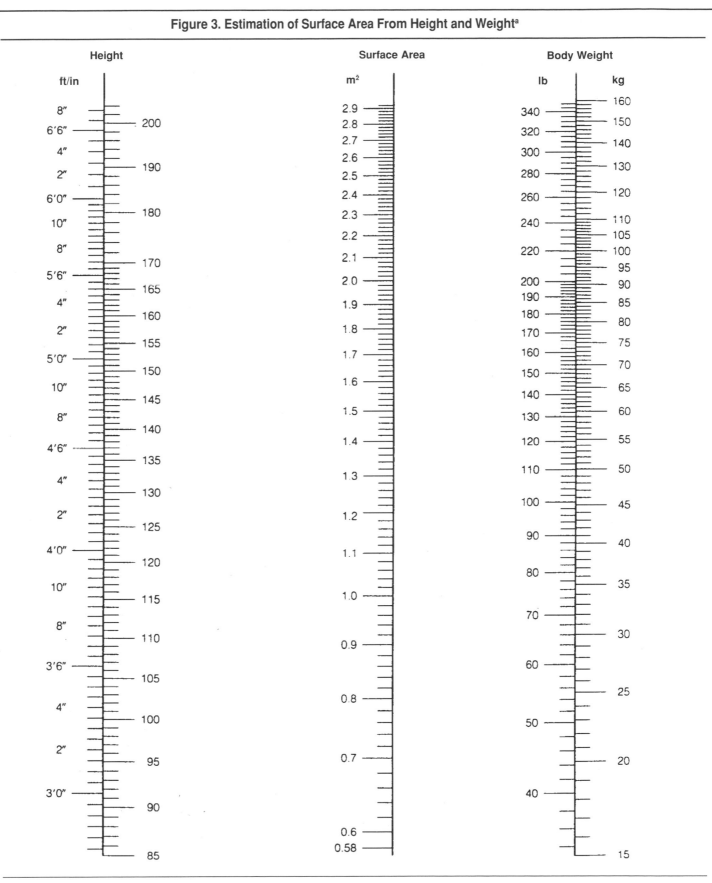

[a] An estimate of a patient's surface area can be obtained by marking the patient's height and weight and drawing a line between these two points; the point at which this line intersects the middle scale represents the patient's surface area.

Note. From *Normal Laboratory Values, Scientific American Medicine* (Vol. 3) (p. 19), by D.C. Dale and D.D. Federman (Eds.), 1996, New York: Scientific American. Copyright 1996 by Scientific American. Reprinted with permission.

(IBW) may be used to calculate BSA. (Refer to an IBW table to calculate IBW per height.) However, if a patient's weight is significantly greater than ideal, average the ideal and actual body weight: (IBW + actual body weight) ÷ 2 (Goodman & Riley, 1997).

    ii) Dose reduction may be required for patients with preexisting hepatic dysfunction, renal impairment, poor performance status, toxicity related to prior chemotherapy, or other comorbid conditions.

    iii) The Calvert formula (Calvert, Newell, & Gore, 1992) is used to calculate area under the curve (AUC) instead of BSA to determine carboplatin dosing. It is based on glomerular filtration rate and plasma concentration. As a result, creatinine clearance is a sensitive parameter to determine drug clearance and bone marrow suppression in patients receiving carboplatin.

(4) Identify appropriate drugs and list expected side effects or toxicities.

(5) Verify that written and/or verbal patient or parental consent has been obtained or that the patient and family understand and are willing to assume the responsibilities of homecare administration (e.g., reporting chemotherapy spills, change in patient condition, change in venous-access status).

(6) Prior to administration of any chemotherapy, assess the patient's previous experience with chemotherapy.

(7) Assess the patient's understanding and readiness to proceed with treatment.

F. Chemotherapy preparation, storage, and transport (Occupational Safety and Health Administration [OSHA], 1995; Welch & Silveira, 1997)

1. The health risk from chemotherapy exposure is measured by time, dose, and exposure route. Main exposure routes include the following.
   a) Absorption through skin or mucous membrane after direct contact, such as during drug administration
   b) Inhalation of drug aerosols or droplets, such as during admixing or changing IV tubing
   c) Ingestion through contaminated food, beverage, or tobacco products
   d) Needle sticks

2. Drug preparation
   a) Follow the manufacturer's recommendations, with attention to solution compatibility, light sensitivity, and stability.
   b) Specially trained and supervised personnel should prepare the drug. The drug preparer will vary in accordance with state nurse/pharmacy practice acts.
   c) Implement policies and procedures that require personnel who may be exposed to airborne particles or aerosols of chemotherapy generated during handling to wear a National Institute of Occupational Safety and Health-approved dust/mist respirator or face mask unless proper ventilation (i.e., class II or III biological safety cabinet [BSC]) is available.
   d) Implement policies that prohibit eating, drinking, smoking, chewing gum or tobacco, applying cosmetics, and storing food in areas where chemotherapy is used.
   e) Train all employees who will prepare or administer chemotherapy in the proper safety procedures and document the occurrence of such training programs.
   f) Include compliance with chemotherapy policy and procedures as part of the quality-improvement program (Maxson & Wolk, 1998).
   g) Distribute chemotherapy drug workloads among the trained personnel to minimize daily exposure (Harrison, 1992).
   h) Although no information is available on the reproductive risks of handling chemotherapy drugs in

workers who use a BSC and wear protective clothing, employees who are pregnant, planning a pregnancy (male or female), or breast feeding or who have other medical reasons prohibiting exposure to chemotherapy may elect to refrain from preparing or administering those agents or caring for patients during their treatment (up to 48 hours after completion of therapy) (Harrison, 1992; OSHA, 1995; Welch & Silveira, 1997). Institutional policies and procedures that support this practice should be in place (Welch & Silveira).

i) Prepare the drug under a class II or class III BSC with vertical laminar air flow.
  (1) Ideally, the hood should be vented to outside with a blower operating continuously, with service maintained according to manufacturer's recommendations (Avis & Levchuk, 1984; OSHA, 1995).
  (2) The hood should be located in a private area with minimal traffic flow to reduce interference with hood air flow.

j) Mixing
  (1) Wear long-sleeve, nonabsorbent gowns with elastic at the wrists and back closure. Use eye protection, masks, and powder-free latex gloves at least 0.007" thick that extend over the gown's cuffs. People with known or suspected latex sensitivity or allergy should use gloves made from an alternate material such as nitrile.
  (2) When opening ampules, clear fluid from the ampule neck, tilt the ampule away from self, wrap gauze or alcohol pad around the neck, and break away from self. A filtered needle should be used to withdraw fluid.
  (3) When reconstituting drugs packaged in vials, avoid aerolization resulting from pressure build-up. Use an 18- or 19-gauge needle and a 0.2 mm hydrophobic filter and create negative pressure in the vial when adding diluent by using dispensing pins or by aspirating the volume of air slightly larger than the volume of added diluent. Slowly add diluent, allowing fluid to run down the side of the vial. Draw the drug into the syringe, checking dose measurement before withdrawing the needle from the vial. Allow pressure to equalize between the vial and the syringe prior to withdrawing the needle.

k) Use a sterile, absorbent, plastic-backed pad on the work area.

l) Label all preparations with patient name and identification number and medication name, dose, route, diluent fluid, volume, and expiration date (Maxson & Wolk, 1998). Label as cytotoxic drugs and dispose of properly.

3. Drug storage
  a) Store chemotherapy drug containers in a location that permits appropriate temperature and safety regulation.
  b) Label all drugs in storage as to their hazardous nature and provide instructions regarding what to do in the event of accidental exposure.
  c) Chemotherapy drug containers should be checked before transport from a storage area to ensure that the package is still intact. Any spillage should be managed according to the agency's (e.g., hospital, clinic) hazardous drug spill policy and procedure. Spill kits should be readily available (see Table 6 and Figure 4).
  d) Chemotherapy stored in the home should be placed in containers that provide adequate protection from puncture or breakage (see Appendix 2).
    (1) Container labeling should indicate the hazardous nature of the contents and provide instructions in the event of container damage.
    (2) Containers stored at home should be kept out of the reach of children and pets and stored in areas free from moisture or temperature extremes. Used containers should be disposed of properly by taking them to

the hospital, clinic, or chemotherapy homecare supplier or through pick-up by a waste-management company.

(3) Spill kits with instructions should be available in the home whenever chemotherapy is present.

(4) Patients and/or family members should be given verbal and written instructions about handling and storing chemotherapy wastes.

4. Drug transport

a) Syringes containing prepared chemotherapy should be transported in a sealed container with the Luer end of the syringe capped off. (Syringes should not be sent with needles in place.) The transport receptacle (e.g., a leak-proof, sealable bag) should be labeled as containing chemotherapy and should be capable of containing spillage if the syringe (vial) is dropped inadvertently.

b) Personnel transporting chemotherapy outside a patient-care area should have spill kits readily available. Should breakage of a container or a spill occur, either in transport or storage, workers should follow their agency's procedures for spill cleanup (Smith, 1987; Welch & Silveira, 1997).

When traveling outside of an agency, additional impervious packing material or leak-proof storage containers should be used to avoid jostling the contents or puncturing the leak-proof sealable bag. Caution also should be taken to avoid temperature extremes. Labels identifying the hazardous nature of the contents should be in plain sight on the outermost layer of the container.

G. Treatment phase

1. General information

a) Only trained individuals should administer chemotherapy.

(1) Always wear gloves when handling the drug, avoid touching it, and wash hands before putting gloves on and after removing gloves.

(2) Wash surfaces that came into contact with the drug with soap and water. Dispose of toweling in a chemotherapy waste receptacle.

b) Explain the procedures for the administration of premedications or other medications, hydration, and chemotherapy.

c) Identify a plan for antiemetic management, including hydration and electrolyte supplementation, if indicated, before, during, and after chemotherapy administration.

d) Designate a workplace dedicated to the handling of chemotherapy.

Table 6. Contents of an Antineoplastic Spill Kit

Number	Item
1	Gown with cuffs and back closure (made of nonpermeable fabric)
1 pair	Shoe covers
2 pair	Gloves
1 pair	Utility gloves
1 pair	Chemical splash goggles
1	Rebreather mask (National Institute of Occupational Safety and Health-approved)
1	Disposable dust pan (to collect any broken glass)
1	Plastic scraper (to scoop materials into dust pan)
2	Plastic-backed absorbable towels
1 each	250 ml and 1 liter spill-control pillows
2	Disposable sponges (one to clean up spill, one to clean up floor after removal of spill)
1	"Sharps" container
2	Large, heavy-duty waste disposal bags.
1	Container of 70% alcohol for cleaning soiled area
1	Hazardous waste label

Note. From *Controlling Occupational Exposure to Hazardous Drugs* (OSHA Instruction CPL 2-2. 20B) (pp. 21-1–21-34), by Occupational Safety and Health Administration (OSHA), 1995, Washington, DC: Author. Copyright 1995 by OSHA.

e) Have a chemotherapy spill kit and chemotherapy waste receptacle readily available.

f) Have emergency drugs and equipment available based on patient history or treatment plan.

g) Use a disposable, absorbent, plastic-backed pad underneath the work area to absorb droplets of the drug that may be spilled inadvertently on the work surface.

h) If the drug is preprepared, check the syringe, bag, or bottle against the original order for accuracy of patient name, identification number, route, chemotherapy agent, dose, volume, infusion time, and drug expiration, based on institutional policy. Prior to chemotherapy administration, double-check everything to prevent chemotherapy errors.

i) Wear a protective gown made of lint-free, low-permeability fabric with a solid front, long sleeves, and tight-fitting elastic or knit cuffs (OSHA, 1995).

j) Put on powder-free, disposable surgical latex gloves. Change gloves after each use, tear, puncture, or medication spill or after 30 minutes of wear. People with known or suspected latex allergy or sensitivity should wear gloves made from an alternate material, such as nitrile, which is relatively impervious to chemotherapy (Jackson, 1995; Lavaud et al., 1995; Welch & Silveira, 1997).

k) Use needles, syringes, and tubing with Luer-lock connectors.

l) Prime all tubing prior to adding antineoplastics, preferably underneath the BSC. If priming occurs at the administration site, the IV tubing should be primed with a

---

Figure 4. Spill Kit Procedure for Home Use

(Please review this procedure with your nurse.)

1. Do not touch the spill with unprotected hands.
2. Open the spill kit and put on both pairs of gloves. If the bag or syringe with chemotherapy drugs has been broken or is leaking and you have a catheter or Port-a-Cath® in place, first disconnect the catheter from the tubing and rinse and cap according to normal procedure before cleaning the spill.
3. Put on the gown (closes in back), splash goggles, respirator.
4. Use spill pillows to contain spill—put around puddle to form a V.
5. Use the absorbent sheets to blot up as much of the drug as possible.
6. Put contaminated clean-up materials directly into the plastic bag contained in the kit. Do not lay them on unprotected surfaces.
7. Use the scoop and brush to collect any broken glass, sweeping toward the V'd spill pillows, and dispose of the glass in the box of the kit.
8. While still wearing the protective gear, wash the area with dishwashing or laundry detergent and warm water using disposable rags or paper towels, and put them in the plastic bag with other waste. Rinse the area with clean water and dispose of the towels in the same plastic bag.
9. Remove gloves, goggles, respirator, and gown and place in plastic bag. Put all contaminated materials, including the spill kit box, into the second large plastic bag and label with the hazardous waste label in the kit.
10. Wash your hands with soap and water.
11. Call the home health nurse, clinic, or doctor's office promptly to report the spill. Plans need to be made to replace the spilled chemotherapy so the treatment can be completed. Arrangements will be made to have the waste material picked up or have you bring it to the hospital for proper disposal.
12. If upholstered or carpeted area is contaminated, follow the above procedure—blot as much of the solution as possible with the absorbent sheets, wash the area with detergent, and follow with a clean water rinse. Do not use chemical spot removers or upholstery dry cleaners as they may cause a chemical reaction with the drug.
13. If the spill occurs on sheets or clothing, wash in hot water separately from the other wash. Wash clothing or bed linen contaminated with body wastes in the same manner.
14. Patients on 24-hour infusions should use a plastic-backed mattress pad to protect the mattress from contamination.

Following these procedures prevents undue exposure and assures your safety. Call your nurse if you have any questions. Thank you.

Note. From "Home Chemotherapy Safety Procedures," by C. Blecke, 1989, *Oncology Nursing Forum, 16,* p. 721. Copyright 1989 by Oncology Nursing Press, Inc. Reprinted with permission.

nondrug-containing fluid or by the backflow method on an infusion pump (OSHA, 1995).

*m)*Administer prehydration and antiemetic premedications. If appropriate, administer medications to prevent hypersensitivity reactions.

*n)*Ensure that the physician's order and approved protocols for the management of extravasation or hypersensitivity reactions are available before administering chemotherapy. Have an extravasation kit or emergency medication available as indicated (see Figure 5 and Table 7).

*o)*Check for blood return and patency.

*p)*Flush the line with a nonchemotherapeutic agent.

*q)*Place a gauze pad under the needle at the y-site during administration in the event of droplets.

r) Properly discard all supplies in a chemotherapy waste container.

s) Monitor for hypersensitivity reactions.

2. Controversies: see Table 8 (Controversial Issues and Arguments Pro and Con for Vesicant Chemotherapy Administration Practices)

3. Peripheral IV

*a)*If the patient has an established peripheral IV site, assess the site for erythema, pain, or tenderness. Avoid using an old IV site greater than 24 hours because it may have less integrity. Check for blood return and fluid flow by aspirating at a y-site close to the IV catheter. Do not pinch the catheter tubing.

*b)*A new IV site for administration of vesicants is preferred but may not be possible (see Table 8).

*c)*If no IV catheter is in place, assess the patient's hands and arms distally to proximally for possible IV insertion sites. Avoid areas of hematoma, edema, impaired lym-

---

Figure 5. Sample Extravasation Kit

Antidote
2–10 cc syringes
2–5 cc syringes
10 cc sterile water
10 cc sterile saline
4–25 gauge needles
4–19 gauge needles
2 x 2 gauze
paper tape
alcohol swabs

Table 7. Emergency Drugs and Equipment for Use in Hypersensitivity/Anaphylactic Reactions[a]

Drug	Strength	Usage
Epinephrine	1:10,000 solution IV 1:1,000 subcutaneous	0.1 mg–0.5 mg IV push every 10 minutes as needed for adults Pediatric dose is 0.01 mg/kg subcutaneous or 0.2 mg–0.5 mg every 10–15 minutes.
Diphenhydramine HCl	25–50 mg	Administer IV to block further antigen-antibody reaction.

Steroids
  Solu-Medrol®[b]
  Solu-Cortef®[b]
  Dexamethasone
	
	30–60 mg
	100–500 mg
	10–20 mg
		Administer IV to ease bronchoconstriction and cardiac dysfunction.

Aminophylline	5 mg/kg	Administer IV over 30 minutes to enhance bronchodilation.
Dopamine	2 mic/kg/min–20 mic/kg/min	Administer IV to counter hypotension.

[a] Additional emergency medications, such as sodium bicarbonate, furosemide, lidocaine, naloxone HCl, and nitroglycerine (sublingual), and emergency supplies, such as oxygen tank, suction machine with catheters, and ambu bag, should be available in case of medical emergency.
[b] Pharmacia and Upjohn Co., Kalamazoo, MI

Table 8. Controversial Issues and Arguments Pro and Con for Vesicant Chemotherapy Administration Practices

Controversial Practices	Pro	Con
Vesicant first	Vascular Integrity decreases over time. Initially, practitioner's assessment skills more accurate. Patient may become more sedated from antiemetics and less able to report burning, pain at infusion site (Otto, 1997).	Vesicant is irritating, compromising integrity of vein. Nonvesicants are less irritating to veins. Venous spasm may occur early during injection, altering assessment of patency (Otto, 1997).
Side-arm administration	Free-flowing IV lines allow for maximal dilution of drugs that could be potentially irritating and provide assessment of vein patency.	Integrity of vein can be assessed more easily and the early signs of extravasation can be noted more easily.
Direct push administration	Integrity of vein can be assessed more easily, and the early signs of extravasation can be noted more easily than with a piggy-back infusion.	
Use of antecubital fossa	Larger veins permit more rapid infusion/administration of drug. Larger veins permit potentially irritating chemotherapeutic agents to reach the general circulation sooner with less irritation to small veins.	Arm mobility is restricted with a needle in place. The risk of extravasation is increased due to patient mobility (e.g., coughing, vomiting). Infiltration could require extensive reconstruction efforts with limited arm use during the healing process, resulting in increased morbidity and decreased function. Because of the subcutaneous tissues, early infiltration is more difficult to assess.
Large-gauge needles (e.g., #19 and #21 scalp vein needles)	Potentially irritating chemotherapeutic agents can reach the general circulation sooner, with reduced irritation to the peripheral veins. Drug administration time is decreased, which reduces the patient's exposure to a potentially stressful environment.	
Small-gauge needles (e.g., #23 and #25 scalp vein needles)	Smaller gauge needles are less likely to puncture the wall of a small vein. Scar tissue may be formed with needle insertion; small-gauge needles cause less scar tissue formation. The patient may experience less pain during the insertion of a smaller needle. Increased blood flow around a smaller bore needle increases dilution of the chemotherapeutic agent. Mechanical phlebitis may be minimized with a smaller bore needle.	

phatic drainage, sites distal to previous IV catheters or venipuncture sites less than 24 hours old, phlebitis, inflammation, induration, or obvious infection. Other sites to be avoided, if possible, include fragile, low-flow, or small veins; sites of previous irradiation; the dorsal aspect of the wrist; and the antecubital fossa. (Heat packs may be helpful in dilating vessels if visualization is difficult.)

d) Insert the IV device (e.g., catheter, winged infusion set) (see *Access Device Guidelines: Recommendations for Nursing Practice and Education,* Camp-Sorrell, 1996).

e) Prior to administering any chemotherapy, flush the line with sterile IV solution and observe for any signs or symptoms of infiltration. Once patency has been established, tape and dress the line in a manner that allows visualization of the insertion site yet secures the needle into place.

4. Drug administration

a) Piggy-back infusion: Check for blood return and IV patency. Insert the connecting tubing into the appropriate primary tubing y-site and initiate the flow rate according to the physician's order. Secure the needle into the y-site with tape or a locking device.

(1) Monitor the patient, particularly during the first 15 minutes, for any signs of hypersensitivity or anaphylaxis. First doses of antineoplastics known to cause hypersensitivity should be administered at a healthcare facility. However, if such drugs are administered in the home, anaphylaxis kits should be available.

(2) Since no documented research for the absolute best method of short-term or bolus vesicant administration exists, vesicants are administered both by piggy-back infusion and IV push. Monitoring for infiltration while minimizing venous pressure with either method often is challenging. Despite the documented lack of re-

search, one should check patency every five minutes for piggy-back infusion, and every 2–3 ml for vesicant IV-push. Depending on the rate or volume of infusion, the schedule of patency checks may need to be readjusted to ensure vein patency.

(3) Vesicants should be administered one at a time unless the protocol stipulates that they be administered simultaneously (Chrystal, 1997).

(4) Administer vesicants only through Luer-lock or other locking connection points to prevent disconnection and possible spillage.

(5) Upon completion of the infusion, check for vein patency and flush the line with a sterile IV solution.

(6) Dispose of supplies in appropriate containers.

b) Continuous infusion: Check for blood return and IV patency. Connect the chemotherapy directly to the IV catheter or as a secondary infusion through a maintenance solution. Ensure that all connections are secure with a locking device or tape.

(1) Vesicant agents that are infused by continuous infusion for more than one hour must be administered through a central access catheter.

(2) Monitor the IV site throughout the infusion as appropriate. Check for blood returns periodically for vesicant drugs. Check exit sites of central line port for signs of infiltration.

(3) Monitor the patient, particularly for hypersensitivity or anaphylaxis if indicated.

(4) When the infusion is complete, flush the line with sterile IV solution.

c) IV push

(1) Check for IV patency. Once patency is established, attach the syringe to the y-site closest to the patient and proceed with administration. When a maintenance solution is used, it should be free-flowing during the infusion of chemotherapy.

(2) In some cases, per institutional practice, nonvesicants may be administered using the two-syringe method.
    (a) Establish IV access and flush the catheter with a saline-filled syringe.
    (b) Remove the saline syringe and attach a chemotherapy syringe.
    (c) Inject the drug at the prescribed rate.
    (d) When the injection is complete, remove the drug syringe and flush the catheter.
    (e) Discontinue the IV, or attach primary IV tubing or an intermittent infusion cap.
(3) Chemotherapy administration rate is based on the drug, the volume in the syringe, and the manufacturer's recommendation. Despite the lack of documented research on the frequency of establishing IV patency during vesicant administration, one should check patency at an interval and using a technique that minimizes venous pressure. Assess patency every 2–3 cc during the administration with gentle aspiration, checking for ease of flow, lack of subcutaneous swelling, absence of pain and burning, and blood return. Smaller syringes (e.g., 3 ml) will increase pressure on the vein (Conn, 1993), so use of a 10 ml syringe is recommended.
(4) Stop infusion if a change in sensation, pain, burning, stinging, or swelling occurs at the IV site or if unable to obtain blood return. Follow the procedure for extravasation if infiltration is suspected.
5. Central venous catheters (CVCs): subclavian catheter, tunneled catheter, implantable port, and peripherally inserted central catheter (PICC)
  a) Verify the type of catheter and placement of catheter tip after the initial insertion and prior to chemotherapy administration.
  b) Subclavian, tunneled, PICC

(1) Inspect the catheter, exit site, and dressing for evidence of leakage of IV fluid. Examine the ipsilateral chest for signs of venous thrombosis (Mayo & Pearson, 1995; Wickham, 1990).
(2) Inspect the exit site for evidence of erythema or swelling and note any complaints of pain.
(3) Aspirate for blood return prior to chemotherapy administration. In the absence of blood return, flush the catheter with saline, gently using the push-pull method in an attempt to obtain blood return. Avoid use of small syringes (i.e., less than 3 ml). If blood return cannot be demonstrated after flushing or repositioning the patient, obtain a physician order for urokinase and proceed with declotting, per the institutional procedure, prior to administering chemotherapy. If unsuccessful, confirmation of line placement through x-rays or dye studies should be established. Chemotherapy administration should be prohibited unless catheter placement and patency can be confirmed (Camp-Sorrell, 1997; Lopez, 1992; Mayo & Pearson, 1995).
(4) If catheter is patent, proceed with chemotherapy administration.
(5) Stop the infusion if an unusual sensation, pain, burning, stinging, or discomfort occurs during administration and follow extravasation guidelines.
(6) When the infusion is complete, flush the line with sterile IV solution.
  c) For implantable (venous, arterial, epidural, peritoneal) access ports:
(1) Confirm the initial line placement using x-ray or fluoroscopy.
(2) Access the port with a noncoring, 90-degree, bent needle (Goodman & Riley, 1997). Needle length should be based on the depth of the port and patient size (i.e., amount of

subcutaneous tissue/fat) to ensure placement in the reservoir.

(3) Establish blood return prior to chemotherapy administration.

(4) Inspect the needle-insertion site for signs of needle dislodgement, leakage of IV fluid, drainage, or edema. Examine the ipsilateral chest for signs of venous thrombosis.

(5) Apply a transparent, occlusive dressing to ensure stabilization of the needle and visualization of the needle-insertion site. Although transparent dressings allow visualization, controversy exists related to the preferred type of IV-catheter dressing (Aly, Bayles, & Malbach, 1988; Hoffman, Weber, Samsa, & Rutala, 1992; Wille, Blusse Van Oud Albas, & Thewessen, 1993). Refer to the Oncology Nursing Society (ONS) *Access Device Guidelines: Recommendations for Nursing Practice and Education* (Camp-Sorrell, 1996) for further study.

d) After drug administration, check for vein patency. Dispose of all supplies in appropriate containers.

e) See Table 9 (Special Tips for Giving Oral Chemotherapy to Children).

f) See Table 10 (Routes of Administration of Antineoplastic Agents).

6. Extravasation

a) Animal studies

(1) Studies performed with animals have demonstrated both effective and ineffective antidotes for extravasation.

(2) Because of anatomical, nutritional, and immunological dif-

Table 9. Special Tips for Giving Oral Chemotherapy to Children

Approach	Problem
Administering oral medications to a child who cannot swallow	Ability to swallow pills is more dependent on the child's past experiences than age. Do not use a medication that has an unpleasant taste (e.g., prednisone) to teach the child how to swallow a tablet.
Tablets	Tablets may be chewed. Crush tablet into fine powder, dissolve in warm water. Mix solution with juice or food acceptable to the child (e.g., ice cream, applesauce).
Capsules	Open capsule (e.g., CCNU, PCB, HU) and sprinkle contents into food. Not all capsules should be opened; consult with pharmacist.
Administering liquid chemotherapy to an infant/very young child	Place liquid in empty nipple, place nipple in infant's mouth, and allow child to suck. Draw medication up into syringe, place along inside of cheek, and administer slowly. Raise child's head slightly during administration to avoid aspiration.
Administering medications with an unpleasant taste (e.g., prednisone)	Discourage chewing of tablets. Mix crushed tablet in juice or food with a strong taste (e.g., peanut butter, maple syrup, fruit-flavored syrup). Mix crushed tablet with a small amount of juice or food. Child must take all to receive total dose. Do not mix with essential food items (e.g., milk, cereal, orange juice). Avoidance may develop through conditioned association. Crush pills and place in gelatin capsule.
Administering partial doses (e.g., 6-MP)	Break scored tablets only. Pharmacy will crush tablets and dispense in unit dose packages. Dissolve crushed tablet in premeasured amount of water; calculate portion that will give correct dose.
Administering oral medications to promote drug absorption	Notify physician if child vomits after oral administration of medication; drug may need to be repeated. (With prednisone, another form [liquid, pill, IV] or oral dexamethasone may be substituted). Control vomiting of oral medications with antiemetics. With single daily doses, administer all tablets at one time to achieve maximum blood level. Some medications should be given between meals on an empty stomach; consult with pharmacist.
Administering oral medications that are irritating to gastrointestinal mucosa (e.g., prednisone).	Give medications with milk or food. Antacids may promote comfort.

Note. From "Cancer Chemotherapy in Children: Nursing Issues and Approaches," by K. Meeske and K. Ruccione, 1987, *Seminars in Oncology Nursing, 3*, p. 122. Copyright 1987 by W.B. Saunders Co. Reprinted with permission.

Table 10. Routes of Administration of Antineoplastic Agents

Route	Advantages	Disadvantages	Potential Complications	Nursing Implications
Oral	Ease of administration	Inconsistency of absorption	Drug-specific complications	Evaluate compliance with medication schedule. Teach patient handling techniques.
Subcutaneous Intramuscular	Ease of administration Decreased side effects	Inconsistency of absorption Requires adequate muscle mass and tissue for absorption	Infection Bleeding	Evaluate platelet count (> 50,000). Use smallest gauge needle possible. Prepare injection site with an antiseptic solution. Assess injection site for signs and symptoms of infection or bleeding.
IV	Consistent absorption Required for vesicants	Sclerosing of veins over time	Infection Phlebitis Extravasation	Check for blood return before and after administration of drugs.
*Intra-arterial	Increased doses to tumor with decreased systemic toxic effects	Requires surgical procedure or special radiography equipment for catheter/port placement; patient lies flat for 3−7 days during drug infusion	Bleeding Embolism Pain	Monitor for signs and symptoms of bleeding. Monitor partial thromboplastin time, prothrombin time. Monitor catheter site. Intense patient education needed for pump and catheter care.
Internal (implanted) pump		Cost-effective only with long-term therapy (i.e., 3−6 months)	Pump occlusion malfunction As above	Specialized nursing education needed regarding arterial pumps.
*Intrathecal Intraventricular	More consistent drug levels in cerebrospinal fluid	Requires lumbar puncture or surgical placement of reservoir or implanted pump for drug delivery	Increased ICP Headaches Confusion Lethargy Nausea and vomiting Seizures Infection	Observe site for signs of infection. Monitor functioning of reservoir or pump. Assess patient for headache or signs of increased intracranial pressure.
*Intraperitoneal	Direct exposure of intra-abdominal metastases to drug	Requires placement of Tenckhoff catheter or intraperitoneal port	Abdominal pain Abdominal distention Bleeding Ileus Intestinal perforation Infection	Warm chemotherapy solution to body temperature. Check patency of catheter or port. Instill solution according to protocol—infuse, dwell, and drain or continuous infusion.
Intrapleural	Sclerosing of pleural lining to prevent recurrence of effusions	Requires insertion of a thoracotomy tube Usually not in nurse practice act to administer	Pain Infection	Monitor for complete drainage from pleural cavity before instillation of drug. Following instillation, clamp tubing and reposition patient every 10−15 minutes x two hours or according to protocol. Attach tubing to suction x 18 hours. Assess patient for pain or anxiety. Provide analgesia and emotional support.
Intravesicular	Direct exposure of bladder surfaces to drug	Requires insertion of Foley catheter	Urinary tract infections Cystitis Bladder contracture Urinary urgency	Maintain sterile technique when inserting Foley catheter. Instill solution, clamp catheter for one hour, and unclamp to drain or according to protocol.

* Specialized nursing education is required for certain administration methods. Refer to individual state nurse practice acts and agency policies and procedures, or see Camp-Sorrell, 1996.

Note. From "Nursing Implications of Antineoplastic Therapy," by C. Bender, in J.K. Itano and K.N. Taoka (Eds.), *Core Curriculum for Oncology Nursing* (3rd ed.), 1998, pp. 641–656. Philadelphia: W.B. Saunders. Copyright 1998 by Oncology Nursing Society. Adapted with permission.

_____

_____

_____

_____

_____

_____

_____

_____

_____

_____

_____

_____

_____

_____

_____

_____

_____

_____

_____

_____

_____

_____

_____

ferences, extrapolation from animal models to humans has limitations.

b) Local reactions from chemotherapy administration
   (1) Definitions
      (a) Extravasation: leakage or infiltration of a vesicant chemotherapy agent into local tissue
      (b) Vesicant: any agent that has the potential to cause blistering or tissue necrosis (Thomas, 1997) (see Table 11)
      (c) Irritant: any agent that causes a local inflammatory reaction but does not cause tissue necrosis (Thomas, 1997) (see Table 11)
      (d) Flare reaction: venous inflammatory response with subsequent histamine release that may result in flare reaction (Curran, Luce, & Page, 1990); incidence is usually about 3% and duration usually less than 45 minutes.
c) Pathophysiology: Tissue damage secondary to drug infiltration damage occurs from one of two major mechanisms (Rudolph & Larson, 1987).
   (1) The drug (e.g., doxorubicin, daunorubicin [Cerubidine®, Chiron Therapeutics, Emeryville, CA]) is absorbed by local cells in the tissue and binds to critical structures (e.g., DNA, microtubules), causing cell death. It then is released into the surrounding tissue. Healing is inhibited as this process repeats itself as the drug is taken up by other cells. Anthracyclines remain active after being released from the dying cells, causing damage to adjacent cells. Application of a cold compress is recommended (Dorr, 1990).
   (2) The drug does not bind to cellular DNA (e.g., vinca alkaloids). Local tissue damage is more readily neutralized. Application of heat is more helpful in this situation (only true for vinca alkaloids, not others).
   (3) Neither heat nor cold benefits some extravasations.
   (4) For DNA intercalators, tissue injury is minimized with conservative management consisting of limb elevation for 48 hours following infiltration in conjunction with ice application for 15 minutes four times daily (Larson, 1985). Heat should be applied instead of ice only with vinca alkaloids. (Heat can inflict further tissue damage if applied to ulcers caused by doxorubicin) (Dorr, Alberts, & Salmon, 1983) (see Table 11).
d) Vesicant infiltration can result in pain, hyperpigmentation, induration, burning, inflammation, sloughing, necrosis, and ulceration (Barton-Burke, Wilkes, Ingwersen, Bean, & Berg, 1996; Dorr et al., 1983, Rudolph & Larson, 1987) (see Photos 1–7). Severe infiltrations may result in damage to tendons and nerves (Wood & Gullo, 1993). Severe tissue destruction ultimately will interfere with the affected extremity's function or lead to the loss of a limb or a breast (Bertelli, 1994).
e) Incidence of chemotherapy reactions
   (1) Vesicant infiltration is documented in 0.1%–6% of patients receiving peripheral chemotherapy, although accurately quantifying it is difficult because of inconsistent documentation and lack of standard nomenclature (Dorr, 1990; Montrose, 1987).
   (2) In a rare review, 21 (6.4%) of 329 patients receiving chemotherapy via implantable ports had extravasation (Brothers et al., 1988). It may result from any of the following causes (Bach, Videbaek, Holst-Christensen, & Boesby, 1991; Dorr, 1990; Wickham et al., 1992).
      (a) Backflow secondary to fibrin sheath or thrombosis
      (b) Needle dislodgement from port

Table 11. Vesicants and Irritants

Vesicants

Chemotherapeutic Agents	Antidote	Antidote Preparation	Local Care	Comments/Nursing Measures
Alkylating agents				
Mechlorethamine hydrochloride (nitrogen mustard)	Isotonic sodium (Na) thiosulfate	Prepare 1/6 molar solution: a. If 10% Na thiosulfate solution, mix 4 ml with 6 ml sterile water for injection. b. If 25% Na thiosulfate solution, mix 1.6 ml with 8.4 ml sterile water.	1. Aspirate residual drug. 2. Use 2 ml for every mg extravasated 3. Remove needle. 4. Inject antidote into subcutaneous (SC) tissue.	1. Na thiosulfate neutralizes nitrogen mustard, which then is excreted via the kidneys. 2. Time is essential in treating extravasation. 3. Heat and cold not proven effective (Dorr, 1990, 1994). 4. Although clinically accepted, reports of the benefits are scant (Ignoffo & Friedman, 1980).
Cisplatin (Platinol®a)	Same as above	Same as above	1. Aspirate residual drug. 2. Use 2 ml of the 10% Na thiosulfate for each 100 mg of cisplatin. 3. Remove needle. 4. Inject SC.	1. Vesicant potential seen with a concentration of more than 20 cc of 0.5 mg/ml extravasates. If less than this, drug is an irritant; no treatment recommended (Dorr, 1994).
Antitumor antibiotics				
Doxorubicin (Adriamycin®b)	None		1. Apply cold pad with circulating ice water, ice pack, or cryogel pack for 15–20 minutes at least four times per day for the first 24–48 hours (Harwood & Govin, 1994).	1. Extravasations of less than 1–2 cc often will heal spontaneously. If greater than 3 cc, ulceration often results (Goodman & Riley, 1997). 2. Protect from sunlight and heat. 3. Studies suggest benefit of 99% dimethyl sulfoxide (DMSO) 1–2 ml applied to site every six hours (Olver et al., 1988; St. Germain, Houlihan, & D'Amato, 1994). Other studies show delayed healing with DMSO (Harwood & Bachur, 1987).
Daunorubicin (Cerubidine®c)	None			1. Little information known. 2. In mouse experiments, some benefit from topical DMSO (Olver et al.).
Mitomycin-C (mitomycin)	None			1. Protect from sunlight. 2. Delayed skin reactions have occurred in areas far from original IV site. 3. Some research studies show benefit with use of 99% DMSO 1–2 ml applied to site every six hours for 14 days. More studies needed (Alberts & Dorr, 1991).
Dactinomycin (actinomycin-D)	None		1. Apply ice to increase comfort at the site. 2. Elevate for 48 hours then resume normal activity. (Goodman & Riley, 1997).	1. Heat may enhance tissue damage.
Mitoxantrone	Unknown			1. Antidote or local care measures unknown. 2. Ulceration rare unless concentrated dose infiltrates (Dorr, 1990).
Epirubicin Idarubicin (Idamycin®d) Esorubicin	None			1. Antidote and local care measures unknown. 2. Cold, DMSO, and corticosteroids ineffective in experiments with mice (Soble, Dorr, Plezia, & Breckenridge, 1987). Esorubicin-phlebitis common (Dorr, 1990).

(Continued on next page)

Table 11. Vesicants and Irritants *(Continued)*

Vesicants *(continued)*

Chemotherapeutic Agents	Antidote	Antidote Preparation	Local Care	Comments/Nursing Measures
Vinca alkaloids/microtubular inhibiting agents Vincristine (Oncovin®e)	Hyaluronidase	Mix 150 units hyaluronidase with 1–3 ml saline.	1. Apply warm pack for 15–20 minutes at least four times per day for the first 24–48 hours and elevate (Larson, 1985; Rudolph & Larson, 1987).	1. Administer hyaluronidase and apply heat for 15–20 minutes at least four times per day for the first 24–48 hours. 2. These two methods of treatment are very effective for rapid absorption of drug (Bellone, 1981; Laurie, Wilson, Kernahan, Bauer, & Vistnes, 1984; Dorr, 1994; Goodman & Riley, 1997).
Vinblastine (Velban®e)	Same as above	Same as above	Same as above	Same as above
Vindesine	Same as above	Same as above	Same as above	Same as above
Vinorelbine (Navelbine®f)	Same as above	Same as above	Same as above	1. Same treatment as vincristine/vinblastine (Dorr & Bool, 1995) 2. Moderate vesicant 3. Manufacturer recommends administering drug over 6–10 minutes into side port of freeflowing IV closest to the IV bag, followed by flush of 75–125 ml of IV solution to reduce incidence of phlebitis and severe back pain.
Taxanes Paclitaxel (Taxol®a)	Hyaluronidase Ice		Apply ice pack for 15–20 minutes at least four times per day for the first 24 hours.	1. Recent documentation of vesicant potential (Herrington & Figueroa, 1997; Ajani, Dodd, Daugherty, Warkentin, & Ilson, 1994) 2. Paclitaxel has rare vesicant potential (probably due to dilution in 500 cc diluent) (Dorr, Snead, & Liddil, 1996). 3. Ice and hyaluronidase have been effective in decreasing local tissue damage in a mouse model (Dorr, Snead, & Liddil, 1996).

Irritants

Chemotherapeutic Agents	Antidote	Antidote Preparation	Local Care	Comments/Nursing Measures
Alkylating agents Dacarbazine (DTIC)				1. May cause phlebitis. 2. Protect from sunlight (Dorr, Alberts, Einspahr, Mason-Liddil, & Soble, 1987).
Ifosfamide Carboplatin				1. May cause phlebitis. 2. Antidote or local care measures unknown.
Nitrosoureas Carmustine (BCNU)				1. May cause phlebitis. 2. Antidote and local care measures unknown.

(Continued on next page)

Table 11. Vesicants and Irritants (Continued)

Irritants (continued)

Chemotherapeutic Agents	Antidote	Antidote Prepraration	Local Care	Comments/Nursing Measures
Antitumor antibiotics				
Doxorubicin liposome				1. May produce redness and tissue edema. 2. Low ulceration potential 3. If ulceration begins or pain, redness, or swelling persist, treat like doxorubicin.
Bleomycin				1. May cause irritation to tissue. 2. Little information known.
Menogaril				1. May cause phlebitis, venous edema, and induration. 2. Increased incidence if concentrations greater than 1 mg/ml infiltrates or administration occurs in more than 2 hours (Dorr, 1994).
Epipodophyllotoxins				
Etoposide (VP-16)	Hyaluronidase		1. Apply warm pack.	1. Treatment necessary only if large amount of a concentrated solution extravasates. In this case, treat like vincristine or vinblastine (Dorr, 1994). 2. May cause phlebitis, urticaria, and redness.
Teniposide (VM-26)				Same as above

[a] Bristol-Myers Squibb Oncology, Princeton, NJ; [b] Pharmacia & Upjohn Co., Kalamazoo, MI; [c] Chiron Therapeutics, Emeryville, CA; [d] Adria Laboratories, Dublin, OH; [e] Eli Lilly and Co.. Indianapolis, IN; [f] Glaxo Wellcome Oncology/HIV, Research Triangle Park, NC

Note. Based on information from Bertelli, G., Gozzo, A., Forno, G.B., Vidili, M.G., Silvestro, S., Venturini, M., DelMastro, L., Garrone, O., Rosso, R., & Dini, D. (1995). Topical dimethylsulfoxide for the prevention of soft tissue injury after extravasation of vesicant cytotoxic drugs: A prospective clinical study. *Journal of Clinical Oncology, 13,* 2851–2855; Lebredo, L., Barrie, R., & Woltering, E.A. (1992). DMSO protection against adriamycin-induced tissue necrosis. *Journal of Surgery Research, 53*(1), 62–65; Rospond, E.M. & Engel, L.M. (1993). Dimethyl sulfoxide for treating anthracycline extravasation. *Clinical Pharmatherapeutics, 12,* 560–561.

(c) Catheter damage, breakage, or separation of a venous access device (VAD)

(d) Displacement or migration of the catheter from the vein

(3) Duration of tissue damage may progress for six months after incident (Rudolph & Larson, 1987).

f) Assessment

(1) Risk factors

(a) Fragile, small, or sclerosed veins

(b) Superior vena cava syndrome

(c) Lymphedema

(d) Peripheral neuropathy

(e) Condition of the patient, medications that produce somnolence or altered mental status, excessive movement, vomiting, coughing

(f) Skill of nurse

(g) Drug administration technique

(h) Site of venous access

(2) Clinical symptoms of extravasation, irritation, and flare (see Table 12)

g) Collaborative management

(1) Management of peripheral extravasation

(a) At the first signs of infiltra-tion, stop administration of the vesicant and IV fluids.

(b) Open the extravasation kit, if available (see Figure 5). Disconnect the IV and attempt to aspirate the residual drug with a syringe.

(c) Notify the physician.

(d) Administer the appropriate antidote, if known, and initiate the appropriate nursing-management measure (see Table 11).

i) If the antidote is administered intravenously, instill the appropriate amount and discontinue the IV catheter, avoiding excess pressure on the site, and then follow policy guidelines.

ii) If the antidote is administered subcutaneously, discontinue the IV catheter, avoiding excess pressure on the site. Inject the antidote (using a 25-gauge needle) into the subcutaneous tissue. Avoid Z tracking, and then follow local care guidelines. The exact administration technique remains unknown.

(e) Instruct the patient to rest and elevate the site for 48

Assessment Parameter	Extravasation		Irritation of the Vein	Flare Reaction
	Immediate Manifestations	Delayed Manifestations		
Pain	Severe pain or burning that lasts minutes or hours and eventually subsides; usually occurs while the drug is being given and around the needle site	Hours–48	Aching and tightness along the vein	No pain
Redness	Blotchy redness around the needle site; not always present at time of extravasation	Later occurrence	The full length of the vein may be reddened or darkened.	Immediate blotches or streaks along the vein, which usually subside within 30 minutes with or without treatment
Ulceration	Develops insidiously; usually occurs 48–96 hours later	Later occurrence	Not usually	Not usually
Swelling	Severe swelling; usually occurs immediately	Hours–48	Not likely	Not likely; wheals may appear along vein line
Blood return	Inability to obtain blood return	Good blood return during drug administration	Usually	Usually
Other	Change in the quality of infusion	Local tingling and sensory deficits		Urticaria

Table 12. Nursing Assessment of Extravasation Versus Other Reactions

hours, and then resume normal activity (Rudolph & Larson, 1987).

(f) Avoid pressure to the extravasation site.

(g) Photograph the extravasation site.

(h) Document the following in the patient record (Wood & Gullo, 1993) (see Figure 6).

  i) Patient name, date, and time

  ii) Needle type and size

  iii) Insertion site, location, and description

  iv) Drug concentration, volume extravasated, and amount of residual drug obtained

  v) Patient symptoms and nursing assessment

  vi) Nursing interventions and patient response

  vii) Physician notification

  viii) Photograph of extravasation site

  ix) Follow-up instructions (see Figure 6)

  x) Nurse's signature

(i) Monitor site at 24 hours, one week, two weeks, and as necessary for pain, redness, swelling, ulceration, or necrosis, depending on the degree of tissue damage. Follow up with serial photographs, if possible.

(j) Consult a plastic surgeon if a large volume was extravasated or if the patient experiences severe pain after the initial injury or if minimal healing is evident two to three weeks after the initial injury (Bertelli, 1994; Scuderi & Onesti, 1994). Follow-up is necessary if pain, redness, swelling, necrosis, or ulceration is present or persists two weeks after the extravasation (Dorr, 1994).

(2) Management of VAD extravasation

(a) If the patient complains of changes in sensation, pain, burning, or swelling at the CVC site or in the ipsilat-eral chest, if a change in the IV flow rate occurs, or if there is no blood return, immediately discontinue chemotherapy and IV fluids.

(b) If the patient has an implanted port, assess the site for proper needle placement.

(c) Aspirate the residual drug, if possible, from the area of suspected infiltration at port pocket or at the exit site of the tunneled catheter.

  i) If extravasation is a result of needle dislodgement in a port, leave the needle in place and attempt to aspirate the residual drug.

  ii) If unsuccessful, remove the needle from the port and attempt to aspirate subcutaneously in the pocket and surrounding tissue (Wickham et al., 1992).

(d) Administer the appropriate antidote, if known, and initiate the appropriate nursing-management measures (see Table 11). Then, follow steps i–x from the "Management of Peripheral Extravasation" section (see left column) (Camp-Sorrell, 1997; Wickham et al., 1992).

  i) If the antidote is administered intravenously, instill the appropriate amount, avoiding excess pressure on the site, and follow local care guidelines.

  ii) If the patient has an implanted port, remove the port needle after instilling the antidote. Inject the antidote into subcutaneous tissue as appropriate and follow local care guidelines.

(e) Collaborate with the physician regarding the need for a radiographic flow study to determine the cause of ex-

Figure 6. Chemotherapy Drug Extravasation Record

Date _____

Time _____

Patient _____

Drug _____ Dilution mg/ml _____

Method of Administration: Piggy Back _____

                               Side-arm _____

                               VAD: Port _____ Tunnel _____ PICC _____

                               Type of needle/size _____

                               Other: _____

Amount infiltrated _____ Amount aspirated _____

Size of infiltration (note size in cm) _____

Location of extravasation

Hand: dorsal surface   *Arm:* ventral surface

hand _____ rt _____ lt _____   forearm _____ rt _____ lt _____

forearm _____ rt _____ lt _____   wrist _____ rt _____ lt _____

wrist _____ rt _____ lt _____   ac fossa _____ rt _____ lt _____

VAD: Describe _____

other _____ Photograph yes _____ no _____

Process Documentation

     Patient symptoms _____

     Assessment of site _____

     Suspected extravasation _____ Definite extravasation_____

     Physician notified: _____ Date _____ Time _____

     Interventions _____ Antidote _____ Cold/warm application _____

Follow-up (document with serial photographs): _____

Patient Instructions

1. Continue with warm/cold compresses for the first 24–48 hours, then as needed.
2. Avoid pressure to the original IV site.
3. Rest and elevate the site for the first 48 hours, then you can resume your normal activities.
4. Call if you experience any of the following.
   - Pain, burning, redness, swelling at the original IV site
   - Skin breakdown or areas of blackness anywhere on skin
   - Difficulty moving hand, wrist, elbow or shoulder
5. Names and numbers to call 24 hours a day

     MD _____

     RN _____

     Other _____

6. Return appointments with _____
     Date/time: _____

Keep main copy in clinical record and duplicate to patient.

Note. From "Delivery of Cancer Chemotherapy," by M. Goodman, in S.B. Baird, R. McCorkle, and M. Grant (Eds.), *Cancer Nursing: A Comprehensive Textbook* (p. 304), 1991, Philadelphia: W.B. Saunders. Copyright 1991 by W.B. Saunders. Adapted with permission.

travasation (e.g., needle dislodgement, thrombosis, catheter damage, catheter migration).

h) Patient education
  (1) Inform the patient and family that extravasation is a possibility with vesicant chemotherapy administration.
  (2) Instruct the patient and family about the importance of reporting immediate symptoms of extravasation and symptoms of delayed reaction.
  (3) Provide written instructions related to extravasation site care and follow-up (see Figure 6).
7. Hypersensitivity and anaphylaxis
  a) Pathophysiology
    (1) Believed to be an antigen/antibody reaction, a type I hypersensitivity reaction that is IgE mediated
    (2) May be related to the nonspecific release of vasoactive substances from target cells/mast cells (Weiss, 1992a, 1992b)
    (3) May be related to the diluent or delivery vehicle rather than the drug
    (4) May be a local reaction or a generalized, systemic response
  b) Incidence: See Figure 7.
  c) Assessment
    (1) Risk factors
      (a) Receiving a drug known to cause hypersensitivity reactions
      (b) History of allergies, particularly a drug allergy
      (c) Previous exposure to the agent

(d) Failure to administer known effective prophylactic premedication
(e) Previous exposure to metals (Ciesielski-Carlucci, Leong, & Jacobs, 1997)
  (2) Clinical manifestations
    (a) Urticaria
    (b) Localized or generalized itching
    (c) Shortness of breath with or without wheezing
    (d) Uneasiness or agitation
    (e) Periorbital or facial edema
    (f) Lightheadedness or dizziness
    (g) Tightness in the chest
    (h) Abdominal cramping or nausea
    (i) Chills
    (j) Symptoms of hypotension
  d) Collaborative management
    (1) Review the patient's allergy history. Record baseline vital signs prior to drug administration.
    (2) Administer premedication as ordered (e.g., corticosteroids, antihistamines, antipyretics) (Bookman, Kloth, Kover, Smolinski, & Ozols, 1997).
    (3) Ensure that emergency equipment and medications are readily available (see Table 7).
    (4) Obtain physician orders for emergency drug procedures before drug administration (Brown & Hogan, 1990; Thelan, Davie, Urden, & Lough, 1994).
    (5) Perform a scratch test or intradermal skin test, or administer a test dose before administer-

Figure 7. Immediate Hypersensitivity Reactions: Predicted Risk of Chemotherapy

High Risk	Low to Moderate Risk	Rare Risk
L-asparaginase[a]	Anthracyclines	Cytosine arabinoside
Paclitaxel	Bleomycin	Cyclophosphamide
	Carboplatin	Chlorambucil
	Cisplatin	Dacarbazine
	Cyclosporine	5-Fluorouracil
	Docetaxel	Ifosfamide
	Etoposide	Mitoxantrone
	Melphalan[a]	
	Methotrexate	
	Procarbazine	
	Teniposide	

[a] Significantly increased risk with IV route

ing the initial dose of drug with incidence of hypersensitivity reactions (e.g., bleomycin in patients with lymphoma).

(a) Observe the patient for a local or systemic reaction, which can occur up to one hour or more after the test is performed.

(b) If no signs of a hypersensitivity reaction appear, proceed with the initial dosing.

(c) When administering an IV bolus drug with an incidence of hypersensitivity, infuse slowly and continue to observe the patient for shortness of breath, flushing, or a change in vital signs.

(d) If a hypersensitivity reaction is suspected, discontinue infusion of the drug, maintain the IV line, administer emergency drugs as preordered, stay with the patient, and have another staff member notify the physician.

(6) Localized hypersensitivity reaction

(a) Observe and evaluate symptoms (e.g., urticaria, wheals, localized erythema).

(b) Administer diphenhydramine and/or corticosteroids per physician order.

(c) Monitor vital signs at least every 15 minutes for one hour and as the patient's condition requires.

(d) Avoid subsequent doses if a patient is considered sensitized to the drug. If the drug is considered critical to the treatment plan, premedication with antihistamines and corticosteroids may prevent a hypersensitivity reaction.

(e) If a flare reaction appears along the vein with doxorubicin or daunorubicin (see Table 12), stop the drug and flush the vein with sa-

line (Curran et al., 1990).

i) If extravasation is suspected, manage as outlined in the "Collaborative Management" section of "Extravasation" (p. 38).

ii) If extravasation is not suspected, continue with a saline flush and observe for resolution of flare (Curran et al., 1990).

iii) If resolution does not occur, administer hydrocortisone, 25–50 mg IV with a physician's order, followed by a saline flush (Curran et al., 1990).

iv) Once the flare reaction has resolved, slowly resume infusion of the drug (Curran et al., 1990).

v) If the drug is to be readministered at a later date, consider premedication with antihistamines and corticosteroids. Slow infusion rates and/or increased dilution of the drug may be helpful.

(7) Generalized hypersensitivity reactions usually occur within 15 minutes of the start of the infusion.

(a) Immediate action is imperative. Many actions may need to be performed simultaneously.

(b) Stop chemotherapy infusion immediately.

(c) Stay with the patient. Another staff member should notify the physician and emergency team or call 911 if indicated.

(d) Maintain an IV line with normal saline or another appropriate solution.

(e) Administer emergency drugs per standing order or physician orders (see Table 7).

(f) Place the patient in supine position.

(g) Monitor vital signs every 2

minutes until stable, then every 5 minutes for 30 minutes, and then every 15 minutes.

    (h) Maintain an airway, assessing for increasing edema of the respiratory tract. Administer oxygen if needed. Anticipate the need for cardiopulmonary resuscitation.

    (i) Provide emotional support to the patient and family.

    (j) Document all treatment and patient responses in the patient's medical record.

    (k) Avoid using the chemotherapy agent that caused the anaphylaxis/hypersensitivity reaction in the future. If the drug is necessary in the treatment plan, the healthcare team should consider the following options.

      i) Medication desensitization with the physician present (Essayan et al., 1996)

      ii) Premedication with antihistamines and/or corticosteroids

      iii) Additional fluid for drug dilution

      iv) Increased infusion time

      v) Substitution of a similar drug (e.g., Erwinia L-asparaginase instead of the *E. coli* form) (Weiss, 1992b)

  (8) Investigational drugs should be administered with appropriate patient monitoring when a physician is available.

  e) Patient education

    (1) Inform the patient of the possibility of a hypersensitivity reaction.

    (2) Teach the patient the signs of a hypersensitivity reaction and to report signs.

    (3) Instruct the patient to inform subsequent healthcare providers of hypersensitivity reactions and the usual premedications administered.

H. Safety precautions

  1. Handling body fluids after chemotherapy administration

    a) Institute universal precautions when handling blood, vomitus, or excreta of patients who have received chemotherapy within the past 48 hours. Wear a gown and goggles when appropriate and if expecting splashing.

    b) Provide a urinal with a tight-fitting lid for male patients (Gullo, 1988).

    c) For children in diapers or incontinent adults, apply a protective ointment to the diaper area to avoid painful chemical burns when voiding. Clean the skin well with each diaper change, and change diapers frequently (Meeske & Ruccione, 1987).

    d) Flush the toilet (septic tank or city sewage) after disposing of body excreta from patients who have received chemotherapy within the past 48 hours.

  2. Linens

    a) Institute universal precautions when handling linens soiled with blood or body fluids.

    b) Linens contaminated with chemotherapy or excreta from patients who have received chemotherapy within the past 48 hours should be contained in specially marked impervious bags. Linens should be prewashed and then added to the hospital or industrial laundry for a second wash (OSHA, 1995).

    c) In the home, wear gloves when handling bed linens or clothing contaminated with chemotherapy or patient excreta within 48 hours of chemotherapy administration. Place linens in a separate, washable pillow case. Wash soiled linens twice in hot water with regular detergent in a washing machine. Do not wash with other household items (Gullo, 1988).

    d) Discard disposable diapers with other hazardous wastes in plastic bags intended for hazardous waste disposal. Cloth diapers should be laundered twice, as should other chemotherapy- or fluid-soiled linens.

    e) After use, discard gloves and gown (if disposable) in a hazardous waste container.

    f) Disposable linens or leak-proof pads should be used for incontinence or vomiting.

g) For further information, see *Safe Handling of Cytotoxic Drugs: An Independent Study Module* (Welch & Silveira, 1997), *ASHP Technical Assistance Bulletin on Handling Cytotoxic and Hazardous Drugs* (American Society of Hospital Pharmacists [ASHP], 1990), and *Controlling Occupational Exposure to Hazardous Drugs* (OSHA 1995).

3. Disposal (Dunne, 1989; Hoffman, 1980; OSHA, 1995)

a) Identify antineoplastic waste products by using leak-proof, sealable plastic bags or other appropriate containers with brightly colored labels indicating the hazardous nature of the contents.

b) Use puncture-proof containers for sharp or breakable items. Needles and syringes must be intact when disposed. Do not break or recap needles or crush syringes.

c) Only those housekeeping personnel who have previously received instruction in safe-handling procedures should handle waste containers. Personnel should be properly dressed in gowns with cuffs and back closure and should wear latex, rubber, or polyvinychloride disposal gloves.

d) Place all supplies used in home chemotherapy administration in an appropriate leak-proof container and remove from the home to a designated area for appropriate disposal by a nurse, patient, or significant other. Make arrangements with the physician's office, hospital, company that supplies medicines and equipment, or private waste-management firm for proper disposal (Blecke, 1989; Gullo, 1988; Sansivero & Murray, 1989). Check county and state regulations regarding the handling of biohazardous wastes.

4. Accidental exposure

a) Appropriate personal protective equipment (e.g., gown, gloves, eye protection, masks) should be worn when participating in the following.

(1) Withdrawing needles from vials

(2) Transferring drugs using needles or syringes

(3) Opening ampules

(4) Expelling air from a drug-filled syringe

(5) Administering the drug

(6) Changing IV bags or tubing of continuous infusion therapy

(7) Being exposed to inadvertent puncture of a closed system

(8) Priming IV tubing with a solution compatible with the chemotherapy

(9) Handling leakage from the tubing, syringe, and connection site

b) Improper technique, faulty equipment, or negligence in hood operation can lead to increased exposure (OSHA, 1995).

c) Acute symptoms of accidental exposure include headache, nausea, dizziness, skin irritation, eye irritation, and throat irritation.

d) In the event of exposure, remove contaminated garment and immediately wash area with soap and water.

5. Spills (see *Safe Handling of Cytotoxic Drugs: An Independent Study Module,* Welch & Silveira, 1997)

a) Spills and breakage should be cleaned up immediately by a trained and protected person (Harrison, 1992).

(1) Don two pair of powder-free latex gloves, a disposable gown, and a face shield. (See page 25 for information regarding latex allergies.)

(2) If airborne liquid or powder is present, a NIOSH-approved respirator should be used.

(3) Liquids should be wiped and absorbed with absorbent gauze pads. Solids should be wiped and absorbed with wet absorbent gauze pads.

(4) Any broken glass fragments should be picked up and placed in a puncture-proof container using a small scoop.

(5) The puncture-proof container, gauze, absorbent pads, and other contaminated materials should be placed into a cytotoxic drug disposal bag.

(6) The spill area should be cleaned three times using a detergent solution followed by clean water.

(7) The cleaning instrument (absorbent pad or towel) should be discarded into the large hazardous waste bag.

(8) Any reusable items used to clean up the spill (e.g., glass scoop) or located in the spill area (e.g., volumetric pump) should be washed twice with detergent and rinsed with water by a trained employee wearing doubled latex gloves, a gown, and goggles.

(9) The large cytotoxic waste bag should be sealed and placed into a second cytotoxic waste disposal bag. Any employees cleaning the spill should remove their protective garb and place it in the outer cytotoxic waste disposal bag.

(10) The outer cytotoxic waste disposal bag should be sealed and placed in a puncture-proof cytotoxic waste disposal container.

(11) Document the following.
   (a) The drug and the approximate volume spilled
   (b) How the spill occurred
   (c) Spill-management procedures followed
   (d) Personnel, patients, and others exposed to the spill
   (e) Notification of appropriate personnel about the spill

b) Spills should be immediately identified with a warning sign so others in the vicinity will not be contaminated (Gullo, 1988).

c) Chemical inactivators, with the exception of sodium thiosulfate (for use with mechlorethamine/nitrogen mustard), should not be used to absorb drug spills because potentially dangerous by-products may be produced (Harrison, 1992).

d) All spills should be wiped up three times with the absorbent toweling available in spill kits (see Table 6).

e) If spills occur on a carpeted surface, absorbent powder should be placed over the spill, not absorbent toweling. Vacuum powder with a small vacuum reserved for hazardous drug cleanup. Then, clean the carpet as usual (ASHP, 1990).

f) All contaminated surfaces should be cleaned thoroughly with a detergent solution and wiped clean with water. Contaminated absorbents and other soiled materials should be disposed of in a hazardous-drug disposal bag (ASHP, 1990).

g) Spills of less than 150 ml volume within BSCs should be cleaned according to the aforementioned guidelines. Spills of greater than 150 ml volume within BSCs require additional decontamination of all interior surfaces once the initial clean-up is complete (Welch & Silveira, 1997).
   (1) Any broken glass should be placed in the puncture-resistant container in the BSC using utility gloves.
   (2) All surfaces of the interior of the BSC, including the drain spillage trough, should be cleaned with a detergent.
   (3) Additional decontamination (using a cleaning agent with a pH of soap that removes chemicals from stainless steel) is necessary when the spill is not contained to either a small area or the drain spillage trough.
   (4) If the spill contaminates the high-efficiency particulate air (HEPA) filter, the BSC should be sealed in plastic and not used until the HEPA filter can be changed by a BSC service technician.

h) Each time a spill of more than 5 ml occurs, a complete record of the spill should be sent to the safety director or a designee of the agency (Cloak et al., 1985; Harrison, 1992).

i) If an oral chemotherapeutic drug bottle is broken, double-bag all of its contents and return them to the manufacturer (Anderson et al., 1993).

j) For spills at home, see Figure 4.

k) Document the spill (i.e., drug, volume, how spill occurred, procedures performed, those exposed).

6. Handling
   a) Agencies must have policies and procedures that protect employees, patients, customers, and the

environment from exposure to hazardous agents.

b) Agencies must have policies and procedures that ensure safe storage, transport, administration, and disposal of hazardous agents.

c) Training programs must be available to all employees involved in the handling of hazardous agents.

d) Agencies should have written policies and procedures related to the medical surveillance of employees involved in the handling of hazardous agents.

e) All employees handling chemotherapy drugs should wear protective clothing, which includes disposable gloves, a gown, and eye protection. All equipment should be removed, and hands should be washed before leaving the work area.

7. Spills—Cleaning

a) Spill kits should be available in all areas where chemotherapy is stored, transported, prepared, or administered. All employees who work in these areas should be trained regarding safe containment of spills.

b) Employees should be advised to report all spills, exposures, or unsafe conditions to their supervisors.

c) Wet mopping or sweeping in areas where spills have occurred should be prohibited until spills have been contained (Harrison, 1992).

d) Once spills have been contained, cleaning should proceed from the least to most contaminated areas. All materials used in the cleaning process should be disposed of as hazardous drugs according to federal, state, and local laws (OSHA, 1995).

I. Documentation (see Appendices 3 and 4)

1. Patient name, date, and time
2. Site assessment before infusion
3. Vein selection, gauge and length of needle inserted, or type of central line
4. Establishment of blood return before, during, and after chemotherapy administration
5. Amount and type of flushing solution
6. Drug name, route, dose, and infusion duration

7. Patient perception or tolerance of chemotherapy administration
8. Post-treatment site assessment
9. Patient education related to drugs received, toxicities, toxicity management, and follow-up care (Otto, 1997)
10. Discharge instructions

J. Ethical issues related to chemotherapy administration

1. Increased ethical concerns have resulted from a number of changes associated with chemotherapy administration.

a) Technological advances: Life-sustaining measures frequently are employed for many reasons, including lack of prior discussions with patients regarding their wishes, reluctance to communicate with grief-stricken families, fear of legal liability, and the historical emphasis on treatment rather than comfort (Marsee, 1994).

b) Cost-containment measures: Cutbacks in nursing personnel, reallocation of resources, consolidation, and corporatization have resulted in growing administrative dominance over clinical practice (Benoliel, 1993).

c) Increasing numbers of uninsured and insufficiently covered individuals: Children and the working poor are most affected by lack of coverage (McCabe, 1993), and some people with coverage are unable to obtain reimbursement for certain treatments, such as bone marrow transplant (BMT) (Barr et al., 1996).

d) Increasing use of unproven cancer treatments: Increasing use, either with conventional treatment or as a substitute for it, is the result of many factors, including the unpredictable nature of cancer and its treatment, the patient's need for control, belief in individuals' rights and determination, and cultural and spiritual beliefs (Fletcher, 1992).

2. Nurses routinely confront ethical issues in daily practice.

a) Ethical issues of concern identified by oncology nurses include end-of-life decisions, informed consent, patient autonomy, right to refuse treatment, undertreatment of pain, healthcare reform, access to care, confidentiality, scientific integrity, and nurse-physician conflicts (Ersek, Scanlon, Glass, Ferrell, & Steeves, 1995; Ferrell & Rivera, 1995; Glass, 1994).

b) Many nurses believe that their educational preparation did not adequately address ethics (Scanlon, 1994) and that, consequently, they lack expertise in ethical decision-making skills.

3. Basic principles of ethical decision making
   a) Autonomy: independent decision making by individuals in accordance with their own best interests
   b) Nonmaleficence: the duty to do no harm
   c) Beneficence: the duty to act in the best interest of the involved person
   d) Justice: equitable distribution of available resources
   e) Veracity: truth telling
   f) Fidelity: faithfulness to promises made
   g) Advocacy: support given to others to assist in their decision-making ability

4. The process of moral reasoning in ethical decision making (Thomasma, 1997)
   a) Six steps
      (1) What are the facts? Research all relevant sources.
      (2) What are the values at risk in the case? Describe the values of the patient, family, physician, staff, institution, and society.
      (3) Determine the principal conflict between values and professional norms or beliefs.
      (4) Determine possible courses of action and state which values and ethical principles each course of action would protect or infringe.
      (5) Make a decision and defend this course of action.
      (6) Evaluate the outcome of the decision on all involved.

5. Ethical issues specifically related to chemotherapy administration
   a) Informed consent

(1) Represents an ongoing process that involves a two-way exchange of information
(2) Necessitates respect for autonomy
(3) Elements of the informed-consent process include competence, disclosure, understanding, voluntariness, and consent (Beauchamp & Childress, 1994).
(4) The informed-consent process is used to obtain consent for treatment, enrollment in clinical trials, and participation in nursing research (Berry, Dodd, Hinds, & Ferrell, 1996).
(5) Nurses and physicians have complementary roles in the informed-consent process (see Table 13).
(6) Informed consent implies the right of the patient to refuse or discontinue chemotherapy treatment. Anecdotal evidence suggests that patients may consent to treatment simply because the physician advises them to do so and that patients may consent with a limited understanding of the risks and benefits involved. Patients fear abandonment when considering terminating treatment and worry about how they will obtain pain relief. Patients refusing treatment should be assured that ongoing support and care will be provided if they decline or discontinue treatment (McGrath, 1995).

b) Phase I chemotherapy research trials
   (1) Assess the safety of agents never before administered to humans
   (2) Strive to define the maximum tolerated dose of a drug through stepwise dose escalation
   (3) Raise ethical questions (Kodish, Stocking, Ratain, Kohrman, & Siegler, 1992).
      (a) Does phase I research sacrifice the individual for the good of society?
      (b) Does the vulnerability of

this group of patients warrant special protection?

(c) Are patients adequately informed about phase I trials?

(4) A study of patients considering experimental drug treatment found that they were subjected to considerable pressure, that they did not ask for more time to think about their decisions, and that they did not seek additional sources of information regarding the proposed treatment and alternative treatments (Tabak, 1995).

K. Legal issues related to chemotherapy administration

1. Healthcare system changes and societal expectations have increased

the oncology nurse's exposure in the legal arena.

a) Technology is advancing.

(1) Increased sophistication of drug-delivery methods (e.g., devices, pumps)

(2) Complex treatment protocols

b) Oncology treatment is shifting from acute-care settings into the community.

c) Patients are "sicker" and being treated "quicker."

d) More nurses have advanced practice roles.

e) Society expects competent health-care providers.

f) The public often equates a bad patient outcome with malpractice.

2. Oncology nursing practice is guided

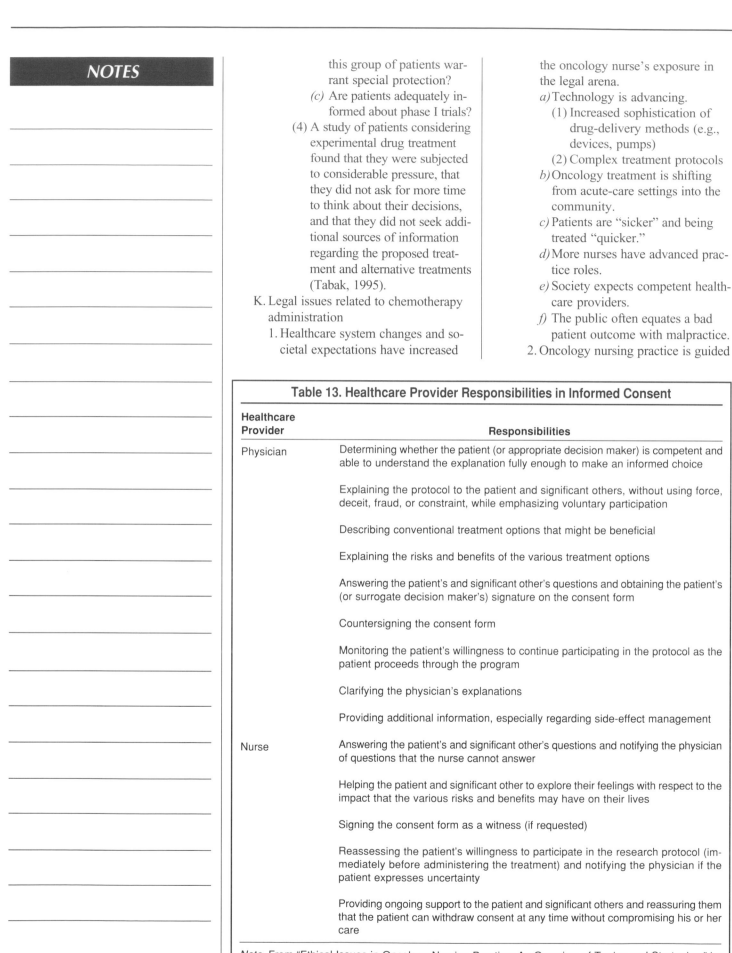

Table 13. Healthcare Provider Responsibilities in Informed Consent

Healthcare Provider	Responsibilities
Physician	Determining whether the patient (or appropriate decision maker) is competent and able to understand the explanation fully enough to make an informed choice
	Explaining the protocol to the patient and significant others, without using force, deceit, fraud, or constraint, while emphasizing voluntary participation
	Describing conventional treatment options that might be beneficial
	Explaining the risks and benefits of the various treatment options
	Answering the patient's and significant other's questions and obtaining the patient's (or surrogate decision maker's) signature on the consent form
	Countersigning the consent form
	Monitoring the patient's willingness to continue participating in the protocol as the patient proceeds through the program
	Clarifying the physician's explanations
	Providing additional information, especially regarding side-effect management
Nurse	Answering the patient's and significant other's questions and notifying the physician of questions that the nurse cannot answer
	Helping the patient and significant other to explore their feelings with respect to the impact that the various risks and benefits may have on their lives
	Signing the consent form as a witness (if requested)
	Reassessing the patient's willingness to participate in the research protocol (immediately before administering the treatment) and notifying the physician if the patient expresses uncertainty
	Providing ongoing support to the patient and significant others and reassuring them that the patient can withdraw consent at any time without compromising his or her care

Note. From "Ethical Issues in Oncology Nursing Practice: An Overview of Topics and Strategies," by G. Winters, E. Glass, and C. Sakurai, 1993, *Oncology Nursing Forum, 20*(Suppl. 10), p. 28. Copyright 1993 by Oncology Nursing Press, Inc. Reprinted with permission.

by several acts and standards (Frank-Stromborg & Chamorro, 1996).

   a) Nurse practice acts: laws that define nursing performance in its most fundamental terms in each state

   b) American Nurses Association and ONS *Statement on the Scope and Standards of Oncology Nursing Practice* (1996): describes the minimum standard of care to which a patient with cancer is entitled

   c) ONS *Statement on the Scope and Standards of Advanced Practice in Oncology Nursing* (1997)

   d) Institutional standards

     (1) Agency policies

     (2) Nursing procedure manuals

     (3) Job descriptions

3. Legal issues related to chemotherapy administration

   a) Chemotherapy medication errors

     (1) Medication administration is considered the most potentially hazardous activity performed by nurses (Medication, Administration, and I.V. Therapy Manual, 1993).

     (2) In review of 12 litigation actions against nurses, 9 cases involved administration of chemotherapy or narcotics in incorrect doses, to the wrong patient, or through the wrong route or extravasation that caused tissue damage (Schulmeister, 1987).

     (3) Chemotherapy errors can be lethal.

       (a) Forty-three deaths were reported to a national medication-reporting database between 1991–1994; 11 of the deaths were attributed to chemotherapy overdoses (Edgar, Lee, & Cousins, 1994).

       (b) The extent of chemotherapy errors is unknown because medication error reporting is based on self-report. Medication errors and errors involving medication devices can be reported anonymously to the Medication Error Reporting Program (call 800-23-ERROR).

     (4) Not all medication errors result in litigious action; caring, professional communication has been shown to be a major reason why some people do not sue, despite adequate grounds for a successful lawsuit (Guido, 1997).

     (5) To be successful in a malpractice cause of action, the plaintiff must prove certain elements to establish liability (Schulmeister, 1998).

       (a) Duty owed to the patient: Was the care provided reasonable, prudent, and comparable to that which a nurse with similar training would provide?

       (b) Breach of duty: Did the nurse's level of care fall below the accepted standard?

       (c) Foreseeability: Could it have been expected that certain events would cause specific results?

       (d) Causation: Is the patient's injury directly related to the breach of the standard of care?

       (e) Actual injury or harm: Did the patient suffer physical, emotional, or financial loss or injury?

     (6) Chemotherapy medication errors can be prevented by employing several strategies, including, but not limited to, the following (Schulmeister, 1997).

       (a) Adhering to institutional policies and procedures

       (b) Verifying chemotherapy doses and schedules

       (c) Using preprinted or computer-generated orders

       (d) Having resources (e.g., reference texts) available

       (e) Reviewing orders and administering the chemotherapy in a nondistracting environment

       (f) Using experienced, certified nurses

   b) Vesicant extravasation (Boyle & Engelking, 1995)

     (1) Patients should be informed of the risks and consequences as-

sociated with vesicant chemotherapy administration in order to detect extravasation at its earliest stages.

(2) The occurrence of extravasation does not imply negligence.

(a) Liability in extravasation-related lawsuits is determined by issues of nursing responsibility for the alleged act, omission of appropriate interventions, or commission of an incorrect intervention.

(b) Critical variables that assist in determining if nursing negligence occurred have been described (Hubbard & Seipp, 1985).

i) Did the nurse adhere to the institution's chemotherapy administration policy?

ii) Was the chemotherapy administered in a prudent and proper manner in accordance with the physician's orders?

iii) Did the nurse stop the vesicant immediately when the patient complained of pain or burning?

iv) Did the nurse exercise reasonable judgment before and during the administration of the vesicant?

v) Did the nurse take appropriate action to manage the extravasation?

vi) Was the physician promptly informed? Was the incident adequately described in the patient's medical record?

(c) The likelihood that an extravasation will result in legal action can be reduced by employing several strategies.

i) Institutionally approved guidelines for extravasation management should be available and reviewed regularly.

ii) A protocol for the management of extravasation should be available prior to vesicant administration.

iii) The patient should be monitored at all times during the peripheral administration of a vesicant by a nurse who has the knowledge and skills necessary to implement the extravasation-management procedure.

iv) The extravasation-management procedure should be initiated as soon as a vesicant extravasation is suspected.

v) Procedures for documenting an actual or suspected extravasation should be defined and followed.

(3) Hypersensitivity reactions

(a) Prior to administration of a chemotherapy agent with known allergic reaction potential, the patient's allergy history should be obtained, and baseline vital signs should be taken and documented.

(b) A test dose of the drug should be administered if applicable and ordered by the physician.

(c) The nurse should ensure that emergency drugs and equipment are available. This is especially important if the chemotherapy is administered in the patient's home or in another nonacute-care setting.

(d) The patient should be instructed to report hypersensitivity symptoms, and this information should be reviewed at each treatment because hypersensitivity reactions can occur with repeated exposure to the drug.

d) Defensive documentation (Schulmeister, 1993)

(1) The duty to keep accurate records is one of the nurse's most fundamental legal responsibilities.

(2) The patient's medical record is scrutinized in the event of litigious action and is believed to reflect the care rendered (i.e., "If it wasn't charted, it wasn't done.").

(3) Common documentation errors include omitting observations of significance, failing to document the patient's response to an intervention, and failing to document patient teaching.

(4) Direct and indirect nursing actions should be documented.

  (a) Telephone conversations, particularly those during which patient instructions or nurse advice is given, should be noted.

  (b) Pertinent conversations with the patient, family, or other caregivers should be documented.

  (c) Interagency referrals should be recorded.

  (d) Patient confidentiality and privacy should be protected at all times.

IV. Symptom Management

A. Myelosuppression
  1. Neutropenia
    a) Pathophysiology (see Figure 8)
      (1) Neutropenia: absolute neutrophil count (ANC) of 1,500/mm^3 or less
      (2) Neutrophils are in the process of constant production and, therefore, are sensitive to the effects of chemotherapy because of their short life span.
      (3) Chemotherapy damages stem cells, thereby decreasing the ability of the bone marrow to replace erythrocytes, neutrophils, and platelets.
      (4) The lowest point in the white blood cell (WBC) count reached after chemotherapy is referred to as the nadir. It most commonly occurs 7–14 days following administration, depending on the specific drugs and dosages. However, with certain chemotherapy combinations, especially nitrosoureas and mitomycin-C, it may take as long as 63 days to reach the nadir.

        (a) Cell-cycle specific agents (e.g., antimetabolites) produce rapid nadirs in 7–14 days with neutrophil recovery within 7–21 days (Barton-Burke et al., 1996).

        (b) Cell-cycle nonphase specific agents (e.g., antibiotics) cause neutropenia in 10–14 days, with recovery at 21–24 days (Barton-Burke et al., 1996).

        (c) Cell-cycle nonspecific agents (e.g., nitrosoureas) produce a delayed and prolonged neutropenia, with nadirs occurring at 26–63 days and recovery at 35–89 days) (Barton-Burke et al., 1996).

    b) Incidence varies according to agents, doses, and administration schedule (Guy & Ingram, 1996).
    c) Assessment
      (1) Risk factors
        (a) Advanced age may contribute to a reduction in bone marrow functioning. Despite the impact of age on overall physiologic function, research has not established that full-dose chemotherapy cannot be tolerated in the elderly (i.e., patients older than age 65), and most studies suggest the opposite (Walsh, Begg, & Carbine, 1989).

        (b) Some patients may be unable to metabolize the drug. Hepatic and renal dysfunction decrease drug metabolism and elimination, causing elevated and prolonged drug blood levels. This will result in increased toxicity (Barton-Burke et al., 1996).

        (c) Limited bone marrow reserves, which cause prolonged neutropenia, may be a result of involvement of the marrow by tumor, which results in prolonged neutropenia (Barton-Burke et al., 1996).

        (d) Malnutrition may decrease the body's ability to repair

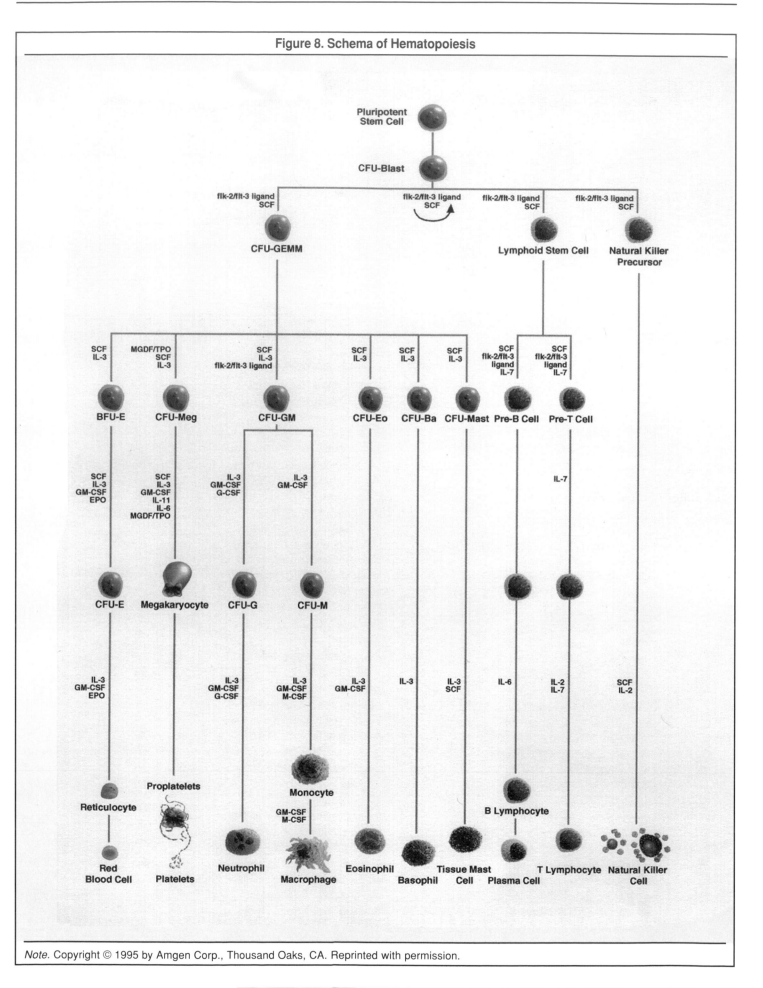

Figure 8. Schema of Hematopoiesis

normal cells destroyed by chemotherapy (Barton-Burke et al., 1996).

(e) Prior chemotherapy may cause bone marrow atrophy or fibrosis.

(f) Concurrent drugs, including antibiotics, antifungals, sulfas, and allopurinol, may inhibit bone marrow recovery.

(g) The risk of infection rises with the severity of neutropenia (see Appendix 1).

(h) Prior radiotherapy of bone marrow-bearing portions of the skeleton, particularly the lower spine and pelvis, has an impact on the resiliency of the bone marrow and may impair bone marrow recovery from chemotherapy.

(2) Clinical manifestations of infection

(a) A fever of more than 38°C or 100.4°F is the most reliable, and often the only, sign of infection in patients who are neutropenic because the body is not producing WBCs, which cause the classic signs and symptoms of infection, such as redness, edema, or pus.

(b) Common sites of infection in patients who are neutropenic and the corresponding signs and symptoms of infection in patients who are neutropenic are the following.

i) Respiratory: Signs include fever, cough, dyspnea on exertion, and adventitious breath sounds.

ii) Skin and mucous membranes: Signs include erythema, tenderness, hot skin, and edema in axilla, buttocks, mouth, perineal, or rectal area.

iii) Urinary tract: Signs include fever, dysuria, frequency, hematuria, and cloudy urine.

iv) Indwelling devices (e.g., VADs, catheters): Signs include erythema, pain or tenderness, edema, drainage, and induration at site.

(c) Septic shock associated with neutropenia has a high mortality rate.

(d) Use laboratory data to assess the degree of neutropenia by calculating ANC.

i) Obtain complete WBC, including differential.

ii) Add neutrophils (polys [segs] and bands).

iii) Convert to percentage.

iv) Multiply total WBC x total neutrophil percentage (polys + bands).

v) Example: WBC = 1,600; polys = 48; bands = 5
  • Add 48 + 5 to get 53
  • Calculate percentage: 53÷100 = 0.53 = 53%
  • Multiply WBC x percent: 1,600 x 0.53
  • ANC = 848

d) Collaborative management

(1) Prevention

(a) To reduce the risk of infection resulting from exogenous organisms, patients often are recommended to avoid exposure to the following. (Note: this practice is controversial and not well-documented in the literature.)

i) Fresh fruits, vegetables, flowers, and live plants

ii) People recently vaccinated with live organisms or viruses (e.g., polio)

iii) Pet excreta, including cleaning of fish tanks/aquariums (because of the potential of fungal and bacterial transmission)

(b) Instruct patients to avoid contact with people who have a transmissible illness (e.g., chicken pox, herpes zoster, influenza, common cold).

(c) People in contact with the patient should be instructed to wash hands prior to touching the patient.

(d) Encourage the patient to practice good personal hygiene through the following.

i) Hand washing

ii) Daily bathing

iii) Mouth care after meals and before bedtime.

iv) Perineal care after voiding and bowel movements (may consider povidone iodine and fresh water sitz baths)

(e) Prevent trauma to the skin and mucous membranes.

i) Avoid catheterizations, enemas, rectal temperatures, and tampons.

ii) Prevent constipation.

iii) Prevent pressure sores.

iv) Use only an electric razor to shave unwanted body hair.

v) Promote healing of all wounds by cleansing and dressing them as directed.

vi) Instruct the patient to use a water-soluble lubricant during intercourse (e.g., Astroglide®, Biofilm, Inc., Vista, CA) and to practice good postcoital hygiene. Intercourse should be avoided during severe neutropenia.

(f) Maintain optimal function of the respiratory system.

i) Encourage the patient to exercise daily as tolerated (e.g., walking, running).

ii) Teach coughing and deep-breathing exercises (e.g., incentive spirometer) to decrease pulmonary stasis, thereby decreasing the potential for infection.

(2) Neutropenic fever management

(a) Culture urine, peripheral blood, all lumens of CVCs, and other suspected sources of infection.

(b) Obtain a chest x-ray.

(c) Perform a physical assessment in an attempt to identify the source of infection.

(d) Administer empiric antibiotics, which should include coverage for gram-positive and gram-negative organisms as ordered.

(3) Follow-up recommendations: When expecting severe neutropenia or planning chemotherapy following neutropenic fever, CSFs may be considered. Refer to Conrad and Horrell's (1995) *Biotherapy: Recommendations for Nursing Course Content and Clinical Practicum* for additional reading.

e) Patient education

(1) Teach the patient, family, and significant other to report the following.

(a) Temperature elevation to 38°C or 100.4°F or greater

(b) Shaking chills (rigors)

(c) Dysuria

(d) Dyspnea

(e) Respiratory congestion or sputum production

(f) Pain

(2) Reinforce the need for meticulous hygiene.

(3) Teach the patient self-administration of G-CSF/GM-CSF as ordered.

2. Thrombocytopenia

a) Pathophysiology

(1) Bone marrow suppression decreases platelet production.

(2) Circulating platelets are diminished gradually because the platelet life span is about 10 days.

(3) Platelets generally recover from the bone marrow suppression after WBCs and before red blood cells (RBCs) (Hoagland, 1992).

(4) Chemotherapy drugs accelerate platelet destruction.

(5) Platelets may abnormally pool to various organs (e.g., spleen) (Fuller, 1990).

b) Incidence
  (1) Chemotherapy commonly induces thrombocytopenia; however, thrombocytopenia rarely has been dose-limiting. More recently, growth factors have allowed chemotherapy dose escalation, which has increased the incidence of thrombocytopenia.
  (2) Incidence varies depending on the agent used.
c) Assessment
  (1) Risk factors
    (a) Radiotherapy or myelosuppressive chemotherapy
    (b) Disease infiltration of bone marrow
    (c) Disseminated intravascular coagulation (DIC)
    (d) Elevated temperature leading to destruction of platelets (Fuller, 1990)
    (e) Drug therapy (e.g., antidepressants, anti-inflammatories)
  (2) Clinical manifestations (Barton-Burke, Wilkes, & Ingwersen, 1992; Tenenbaum, 1989)
    (a) Petechiae, bruising, and hemorrhage (skin, gastrointestinal, genitourinary).
    (b) Neurological signs (e.g., headache, confusion, somnolence), which may indicate intracranial bleeding
    (c) Hypotension and tachycardia
  (3) Laboratory indicators
    (a) Risk of bleeding is present when platelet count falls below 50,000/mm^3
      i) High risk: less than 20,000/mm^3
      ii) Critical risk: less than 10,000/mm^3
    (b) Hemoglobin (Hgb) and hematocrit (Hct)
    (c) Assessment of coagulation tests (e.g., prothrombin time, activated partial thromboplastin time, thrombin time, platelet aggregation) to determine if patient has DIC.
d) Collaborative management
  (1) Activity
    (a) Institute bleeding precau-

tions when platelet count is less than 50,000/mm^3.
    (b) Decrease activity to prevent injury (e.g., falls, bumping into objects).
    (c) Maintain safe environment (e.g., non-skid rugs on floor)
    (d) Discourage the patient from heavy lifting and performing Valsalva maneuvers, which may increase the risk of intracranial hemorrhage (Wroblewski & Wroblewski, 1981).
  (2) Nutrition: Encourage the patient to eat a high-fiber diet and to drink adequate fluids to prevent constipation.
  (3) Daily care
    (a) Instruct the patient to avoid using straight-edge razors and to use an electric razor.
    (b) Instruct the patient to avoid using nail clippers and to use a nail file.
    (c) Avoid administering vaginal douches, rectal suppositories, and enemas.
    (d) Instruct the patient to use a water-soluble lubricant for sexual intercourse (vaginal or anal) and to avoid intercourse when platelet count is severely low (less than 50,000/mm^3).
    (e) Instruct menstruating women to monitor their pad count and amount of saturation. Tampons should be avoided.
    (f) Encourage the patient to blow his or her nose gently.
    (g) Instruct the patient to avoid dental floss and oral irrigators (e.g., WaterPik®, Teledyne WaterPik, Fort Collins, CO) and to use a soft toothbrush or sponge-tipped applicator for mouth care.
  (4) Medications/treatments
    (a) Maintain systolic blood pressure at less than 140 mm/Hg to prevent increased intracranial pressure.

(b) Administer stool softeners or laxatives to avoid constipation.

(c) Avoid nonsteroidal anti-inflammatory drugs (NSAIDs) and aspirin-containing drugs because most alter platelet aggregation.

(d) Avoid intramuscular injections.

(e) Apply pressure 5-10 minutes following venipuncture, bone marrow biopsy, and other necessary invasive procedures. (Platelet transfusion may be required for invasive procedures if platelet count is less than or equal to 50,000 mm³ [Stehling et al., 1994].)

(f) Administer low-dose corticosteroids as ordered for transient thrombocytopenia (Hoagland, 1992).

(g) Administer platelets prophylactically when the platelet count is less than 10,000-20,000/mm³ or if the patient shows signs of bleeding. (Some centers transfuse platelets at 5,000/mm³ if the patient is afebrile and nonbleeding [Beutler, 1993; Stehling et al., 1994].) Institutional policies should be consulted for specific parameters for platelet transfusion.

i) Administer single-donor platelets to patients without alloimmunization.

ii) Cross-matched platelets should be considered for refractory or alloimmunized patients and are the best same-day source of platelets for the patient who is alloimmunized.

iii) Administer human leukocyte antigen (HLA)-matched platelets for patients who are highly refractory, alloimmunized, or multitransfused.

iv) Administer cytomegalovirus (CMV)-negative and irradiated cross-matched platelets to potential BMT recipients.

(h) Prevent transfusion reactions.

i) Infuse leukocyte-poor platelets

ii) Premedicate the patient with an antihistamine, acetaminophen, and/or steroid to prevent transfusion reactions as ordered.

(i) Consider IV meperidine (Demerol®, Sanofi Winthrop Pharmaceuticals, New York, NY) for rigors related to platelet transfusion reactions (Fuller, 1990).

(j) Some newer hematopoietic CSFs (e.g., interleukin-2, and, most recently, thrombopoietin [e.g., oprelvekin, Neumega®, Genetics Institute, Cambridge, MA]) are associated with platelet (megakaryocyte) stimulation.

e) Patient education

(1) The patient should immediately notify the nurse or physician of symptoms of bleeding.

(2) Instruct the patient about the signs of transfusion reaction.

(3) Teach the patient to test urine and stool for occult blood.

(4) See the recommendations under "Anemia."

Anemia

a) Pathophysiology

(1) Bone marrow suppression: suppression of the stem cell or interference with cell proliferation by chemotherapy agents; includes erythrocyte-proliferation pathways

(2) Alteration in erythroblast development

(a) DNA cell-cycle specific agents inhibit the overall production of DNA, resulting in the alteration of erythrocyte development.

(b) Cytoplasmic maturation exceeds nuclear maturation (Hoagland, 1992).

(3) Peripheral macrocytosis: increase in the size of erythrocytes resulting from megaloblastic changes in the bone marrow following chemo-

therapy administration, particularly methotrexate (folic-acid depletion) (Hoagland, 1992)

(4) Kidney damage resulting in reduced production of erythropoietin, especially after large cumulative cisplatin doses

b) Incidence

(1) The degree of anemia is related to drug, dose, and length of treatment regimens. Severe anemia rarely occurs from chemotherapy alone.

(2) Anemia occurs later than neutropenia and thrombocytopenia because the life span of RBCs is considerably longer (120 days) than that of WBCs (neutrophils 4 days) and platelets (10 days) (Hoagland, 1992).

(3) Macrocytosis is common with long-term hydroxyurea and usually is noted by mean corpuscular volumes of more than 115 mm^3.

c) Assessment

(1) Risk factors

(a) Specific drug, cumulative chemotherapy, or high-dose chemotherapy (e.g., cisplatin)

(b) Tumor infiltration of the bone marrow resulting in decreased RBC precursors

(c) Prior or concomitant radiation exposure to bone marrow with associated fibrosis, especially in sternum, long bones, and sacrum

(d) Active bleeding or hemorrhaging (Barton-Burke et al, 1996).

(e) Age

i) Younger patients are more tolerant of chemotherapy because their marrow is more cellular and has a lower percentage of fat (Hoagland, 1992).

ii) Elderly patients may experience delayed marrow recovery resulting from declining physiologic function (Blesch, 1988).

(f) Nutrition: Patients with a negative nitrogen balance (e.g., BMT recipients) and associated weight loss are unable to tolerate anemia because of the potential inability to repair cells damaged by chemotherapy.

(g) Metabolism: Renal and hepatic dysfunction may result in prolonged blood levels of drug and increased marrow toxicity (Creaven & Mihich, 1977; Dewys et al., 1980).

(2) Clinical manifestations (see Table 14)

d) Collaborative management

(1) Encourage the patient to rest to conserve energy.

(2) Encourage the patient to change positions slowly to prevent dizziness secondary to postural hypotension.

(3) Administer oxygen therapy when oxygen saturation is less than 90% or when the patient is symptomatic.

(4) Instruct the patient to eat a diet high in iron (e.g., green, leafy vegetables, liver, red meats).

(5) Administer iron supplements as ordered (Dodd, 1991).

(6) Transfuse RBCs as ordered.

(a) Premedicate with an antipyretic and/or antihistamine per physician order to prevent antibody reaction, and provide comfort from associated fever (Tenenbaum, 1989).

(b) Potential BMT recipients or patients with demonstrable leukoagglutinins should be transfused with leukocyte-poor, irradiated, or frozen RBCs (Barton-Burke et al., 1996; Hoagland, 1992).

(c) Administering leukocyte-poor RBCs is especially important if the patient has previously received numerous RBC transfusions (Hoagland, 1992). Removal of leukocytes from RBCs can be obtained by using leukocyte removal filters during administration or by the blood bank at the time of preparation.

(7) Administer rHu erythropoietin alfa as ordered.

   (a) Patient selection: Hct of less than 30% or Hgb of less than 9 g/dL and one of the following:

      i) Patient is receiving radiation and/or chemotherapy.

      ii) Patient's bone marrow is infiltrated by tumor.

      iii) Patient has a myelodysplastic syndrome.

      iv) Transferrin saturation is at least 20%.

      v) Serum ferritin level is greater than 100 ng/ml.

   (b) Dosing criteria (Ortho Biotech Corporation, 1994; Oster et al., 1990; Symann, 1991)

      i) 150µ/kg SQ/IV is administered three times a week, or the total weekly dose may be divided to be administered daily over five to seven days, or 40,000µ/kg can be administered every week.

      ii) A response usually occurs after two to four weeks, evidenced by an increase in Hct and reticulocytes.

      iii) If the Hct increases by more than 4% in any two-week period, decrease the dose by 50%. If the Hct is not increased by 5%–6% within four to six weeks, increase the dose by 50%.

      iv) Maximum dose is 300µ/kg three times a week.

   (c) Monitoring

      i) After initiation of rHu erythropoietin alfa therapy, monitor Hct at least weekly until it reaches 30%.

      ii) Once a therapeutic dose has been established, monitor Hct at least monthly. Therapy should be discontinued when it is 36% or greater

or when Hgb is 12 g/dL or greater.

   d) Patient education

     (1) Instruct the patient on signs and symptoms of anemia and when to report to nurse or physician (see Table 14).

     (2) Instruct the patient on self-management of the symptoms of anemia.

     (3) Instruct the patient on self-injection of rHu erythropoietin alfa when indicated (Shaffer, 1994).

B. Gastrointestinal/mucosal

  1. Nausea and vomiting

    a) Pathophysiology

      (1) Definitions: Nausea, retching, and vomiting are independent phenomena that can occur sequentially or as separate entities.

        (a) Nausea is the conscious recognition of the imminent need to vomit and may or may not result in vomiting.

        (b) Retching, also known as "dry heaves," is a rhythmic contraction of the respiratory and abdominal muscles, which may or may not accompany vomiting.

        (c) Vomiting is the forceful expulsion of gastric contents through the mouth.

      (2) Mechanisms of emesis

        (a) Most acute chemotherapy-related nausea and vomiting is initiated by stimulation of the vagus nerve by serotonin (5-HT$_3$) released by enterochromaffin cells in the upper gastrointestinal tract (Cubeddu, 1992; Perez, 1995).

        (b) The chemoreceptor trigger zone (CTZ), located in the lateral reticular formation of the medulla, may play a role in acute and delayed nausea and vomiting (Mitchell & Schein, 1982).

        (c) Afferent pathways from the gastrointestinal viscera, the CTZ, the midbrain, the cerebral cortex, and the vestibular system stimulate

the emetic center or the true vomiting center (TVC) to produce the act of vomiting (Hesketh & Gandara, 1991; Mitchell & Schein, 1982).

(d) The TVC initiates impulses to the salivary, vasomotor, and respiratory centers and the cranial nerves, which send somatic and visceral efferents to stimulate the abdominal muscles, the diaphragm, the stomach, and the esophagus in the act of vomiting.

(e) Diaphragmatic and abdominal muscles contract and increase gastric pressure, and gastric contents are released as the gastroesophageal sphincter relaxes (Friedman & Isselbacher, 1991; Pervan, 1990) (see Figure 9).

(3) Patterns of therapy-related emesis

(a) Anticipatory: conditioned response resulting from repeated association of chemotherapy-induced nausea and vomiting and stimulus from the environmental cues surrounding treatment (Andrykowski, 1988);

Table 14. Clinical Manifestations of Anemia

Manifestation	Normal	Mild Anemia	Severe Anemia
Hemoglobin level (mg/dl)	14–18 (M) 12–16 (F)	8–12 mg/dl	< 8 mg/dl
Hematocrit level (%)	42–52 (M) 37–47 (F)	31%–37%	< 25%
Associated symptoms		Pallor Fatigue Slight dyspnea Palpitation Sweating on exertion	Headache Dizziness Irritability Dyspnea on exertion and at rest Angina Compensatory tachycardia Tachypnea
General		Fatigue—often asymptomatic	Fatigue Exercise intolerance
Central nervous system			Dizziness Headaches Irritability Difficulty sleeping Difficulty concentrating
Cardiovascular		Tachycardia Palpitations with exertion	Tachycardia Palpitations at rest Systolic ejection murmur S_3 (extra heart sound)
Pulmonary		Dyspnea with exertion	Dyspnea at rest
Gastrointestinal			Anorexia Indigestion
Genitourinary			Menstrual problems Male impotence
Skin			Pallor Sensitivity to cold

Note. From "A New Approach to Managing Chemotherapy-Related Anemia: Nursing Implications of Epoetin Alfa," by P.T. Rieger and D. Haeuber, 1995, *Oncology Nursing Forum, 22*, p. 73. Copyright 1995 by Oncology Nursing Press, Inc. Adapted with permission.

most commonly associated with cisplatin-containing regimens

(b) Acute: occurs 0–24 hours after chemotherapy administration

(c) Delayed: persists one to four days after chemotherapy administration (mechanisms not well-defined)

b) Incidence

(1) Incidence depends upon the emetic potential of the drugs and the administration schedule used (see Table 15).

(2) Nitrogen mustard and cisplatin (greater than 100 mg/m^2) are the most emetogenic (Mitchell & Schein, 1982).

(3) Administration of high-dose agents, especially alkylating agents, increases the incidence and severity of nausea and vomiting.

c) Assessment

(1) Risk factors

(a) Females have a higher incidence than males (Tonato et al., 1993).

(b) Younger patients experience more nausea and vomiting than their older counterparts (Redd, Burish, & Andrykowski, 1985).

(c) Concomitant medications, such as narcotics and antibiotics, may cause nausea and/or vomiting.

Figure 9. Pathways of Nausea and Vomiting

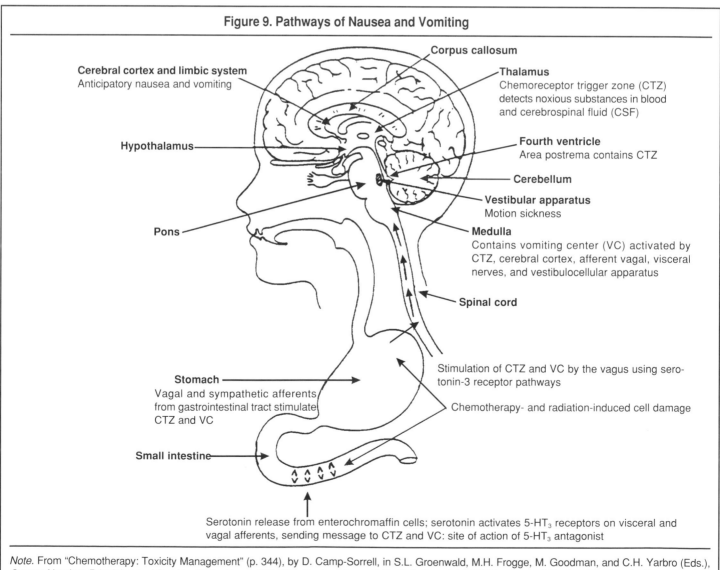

Corpus callosum

Cerebral cortex and limbic system
Anticipatory nausea and vomiting

Thalamus
Chemoreceptor trigger zone (CTZ) detects noxious substances in blood and cerebrospinal fluid (CSF)

Hypothalamus

Fourth ventricle
Area postrema contains CTZ

Cerebellum

Vestibular apparatus
Motion sickness

Pons

Medulla
Contains vomiting center (VC) activated by CTZ, cerebral cortex, afferent vagal, visceral nerves, and vestibulocellular apparatus

Spinal cord

Stomach
Vagal and sympathetic afferents from gastrointestinal tract stimulate CTZ and VC

Stimulation of CTZ and VC by the vagus using serotonin-3 receptor pathways

Chemotherapy- and radiation-induced cell damage

Small intestine

Serotonin release from enterochromaffin cells; serotonin activates 5-HT$_3$ receptors on visceral and vagal afferents, sending message to CTZ and VC: site of action of 5-HT$_3$ antagonist

Note. From "Chemotherapy: Toxicity Management" (p. 344), by D. Camp-Sorrell, in S.L. Groenwald, M.H. Frogge, M. Goodman, and C.H. Yarbro (Eds.), *Cancer Nursing: Principles and Practice* (3rd ed.), pp. 331–365. Boston: Jones & Bartlett. Copyright 1993 by Jones & Bartlett. Reprinted with permission.

(d) Anxiety, pain, expectations, or previous experiences may influence the incidence and severity of nausea and vomiting and the response to ameliorative measures.

(e) Dehydration may accelerate nausea and vomiting (Pervan, 1990; Pisters & Kris, 1992; Wickham; 1989).

(f) A history of motion sickness may predispose some to experience chemotherapy-related nausea or vomiting (Jacobsen et al., 1988).

(g) Patients with a history of nausea and vomiting with previous chemotherapy are at greater risk of developing anticipatory nausea and/or vomiting.

(h) History of nausea and vomiting unrelated to chemotherapy (e.g., morning sickness) may predispose some to experience chemotherapy-related nausea and vomiting.

(i) Change in taste sensations during therapy often produces anorexia and nausea (Pickett, 1991).

(2) Additional assessment

(a) Rule out etiologies other than cancer therapies

Table 15. Emetogenic Potential, Onset, and Duration of Select Chemotherapeutic Agents

Incidence	Agent	Onset (Hours) Nausea and Vomiting	Duration (Hours) Nausea and Vomiting
Very high (>90%)	Cisplatin[a]	1–6	24–72+
	Dacarbazine	1–3	1–12
	Mechlorethamine	0.5–2	8–24
	Melphalan (high dose)	3–6	6–12
	Dactinomycin or actinomycin D	1–2	4–20
High (60%–90%)	Carmustine[a]	2–4	4–24
	Cyclophosphamide[b]	4–12	12–24
	Procarbazine	24–27	Variable
	Etoposide[b]	4–6	24+
	Methotrexate[a]	1–12	24–72
	Cisplatin[a]	1–6	24–72+
Moderate (30%–60%)	Doxorubicin	4–6	6+
	Mitoxantrone	4–6	6+
	5-Fluorouracil[a]	3–6	24+
	Mitomycin-C[a]	1–4	48–72
	Carboplatin[a]	4–6	12–24
	Ifosfamide	3–6	24–72
	Cytarabine[a]	6–12	3–12
Low (10%–30%)	Bleomycin	3–6	—
	Daunorubicin[a]	1–2	—
	Etoposide[b]	3–8	—
	Melphalan[a]	6–12	—
	6-Mercaptopurine	4–8	—
	Methotrexate[a]	4–12	3–12
	Mitomycin-C[a]	1–4	48–72
	Vinblastine	4–8	—
	Lomustine[a]	2–6	2–24
Very low (<10%)	Vincristine	4–8	—
	Chlorambucil	48–72	—
	Paclitaxel	4–8	—

[a] Dose related; potential increases with higher doses.

[b] Route and dose related

Note. From "Chemotherapy: Toxicity Management" (p. 346), by D. Camp-Sorrell, in S.L. Groenwald, M.H. Frogge, M. Goodman, and C.H. Yarbro (Eds.), *Cancer Nursing: Principles and Practice* (3rd ed.), pp. 331–365. Boston: Jones & Bartlett. Copyright 1993 by Jones & Bartlett. Adapted with permission.

(e.g., bowel obstruction, infection, metabolic abnormalities, hepatic dysfunction, increased intracranial pressure, and medications such as opioids).

(b) Nausea and vomiting associated with the tumor (e.g., bowel obstruction, metabolic abnormalities) may decrease after the tumor is treated.

(3) Potential complications of nausea and vomiting (Wickham, 1989)

(a) Patient discomfort

(b) Noncompliance with treatment

(c) Interference with treatment

(d) Dehydration

(e) Increased antineoplastic toxicity

(f) Metabolic disturbances

(g) Anorexia and weight loss

d) Collaborative management

(1) Pharmacologic (see Table 16)

(a) Choose antiemetics that are appropriate to the antineoplastic agent and the dose administered.

(b) Administer antiemetics to cover the expected emetogenic period of the antineoplastic, considering duration and pattern of emesis.

(c) Provide alternative antiemetics to manage breakthrough nausea and vomiting, considering other pharmacologic factors (e.g., maximal binding to 5-HT$_3$ receptors, role of other neurotransmitters).

(d) Dexamethasone is believed to be the most active antiemetic agent in managing anticipatory nausea and vomiting (Cleri, 1995).

(e) IV fluids

(2) Psychosocial

(a) Provide emotional support through counseling and behavioral therapies (e.g., relaxation, progressive muscle relaxation, hypnosis) (Cotanch, 1991).

(b) Other approaches, such as distraction with music, art, or exercise, also may help

to decrease nausea (Winningham & Mac-Vicar, 1988).

(3) Dietary

(a) Encourage the patient to eat small, frequent meals.

(b) Recommend a clear-liquid diet during acute episodes (Tenenbaum, 1989).

(c) Encourage the patient to avoid sweet, fatty, salty, or spicy foods.

(d) Determine foods the patient has used in the past to decrease nausea (e.g., carbonated drinks, crackers).

(4) Follow-up recommendations: Contact the patient 24–48 hours post-treatment to assess control of nausea and vomiting.

e) Patient education

(1) Instruct the patient to notify the staff if nausea and vomiting persist for more than 24 hours or if he or she is unable to maintain a fluid intake.

(2) Instruct the patient to maintain an antiemetic schedule at home for 48–72 hours to avoid delayed nausea. This is indicated for patients receiving cisplatin, high-dose chemotherapy, or highly emetogenic combinations (e.g., CAF; mechlorethamine, vincristine, procarbazine [Matulane®, Roche Laboratories, Nutley, NJ], and prednisone [MOPP]).

2. Diarrhea

a) Pathophysiology

(1) Chemotherapy affects cells with rapid turnover, such as the villi and microvilli of the gastrointestinal mucosa. Chemotherapy drugs most commonly associated with diarrhea are antimetabolites. However, other antineoplastic drugs also may cause diarrhea (Basch, 1987; Mitchell & Schein, 1982; Slichenmyer, Rowinsky, Donehower, & Kaufmann, 1993).

(a) Irinotecan (Camptosar®, Pharmacia and Upjohn Inc., Kalamazoo, MI)

(b) Fluorouracil

Table 16. Antiemetic Therapy: Select Pharmacologic Agents for the Control of Chemotherapy-Induced Nausea and Vomiting

Classification	Generic Name	Trade Name(s)	Route	Dose/Schedule	Duration of Action	Adverse Events
Serotonin antagonist	Ondansetron	Zofran®[a]	IV	0.15 mg/kg, Q4H x 3 doses or 32 mg, 30 min. prechemotherapy x 1	half life = 3–4 hours	Headache, diarrhea, constipation, fever, transient increases in serum SGOT/SGPT
			PO	8 mg BID x 3 days	PO bioavailability 60%	
	Granisetron	Kytril®[b]	IV	10 mcg/kg over 5 min., within 30 min. of chemotherapy	half life = 8–10 hours	Headache, asthenia, diarrhea, constipation, fever, somnolence
			PO	1 mg BID		
	Dolasetron	Anzemet®[c]	PO	100 mg, one hour prechemotherapy	Peak: 1 hour	Headache, diarrhea, dizziness, fatigue, abnormal liver functions
			IV	1.8 mg/kg, 30 min. prechemotherapy, or fixed doses of 100 mg	Peak: 30 min	
Substituted benzamide	Metoclopramide	Reglan®[d]	IV	2.0–4.0 mg/kg Q2H x 4	Onset: 1–30 min. half life = 8–10 hours, Duration: 2 hours	Sedation, akathisia, acute dystonic reactions (increased incidence in patients < 30 years), diarrhea (high doses), dry mouth
			PO	0.5–2.0 mg/kg Q3–4H	Onset: 0.5–1 hour, Duration: 1–2 hours	
Phenothiazines	Prochlorperazine	Compazine®[b]	IM	10 mg Q3–4H	Onset: 10–20 min. Duration: 3–12 hours	Sedation, akathisia, extrapyramidal reactions, dry mouth, orthostatic hypotension, blurred vision
			IV	10–40 mg Q3–4H	Onset: 10–20 min. Duration: 3–4 hours	
			PO	10 mg Q4–6H	Onset: 30–40 min. Duration: 3–4 hours	
			Spansule	15–30 mg Q12H	Onset: 30–40 min. Duration: 10–13 hours	
			PR	25 mg Q4–6H	Onset: 60 min. Duration: 3–4 hours	
	Chlorpromazine	Thorazine®[b]	IM	12.5–50 mg Q4–6H	Onset: 15–30 min. Duration: 12 hours	Sedation, hypotension, dizziness, akathisia, extrapyramidal reactions, dry mouth
			IV	12.5–50 mg Q4–6H	Onset: 5 min.	
			PR	12.5–50 mg Q4–6H	Onset: erratic	
	Perphenazine	Trilafon®[e]	PO	4 mg Q4–6H	Onset: erratic, Peak: 2–4 hours	Sedation, constipation, extrapyramidal reactions, dry mouth, rash
			IM	5 mg Q4H	Onset: 10 min. Duration: 6 hours	
			IV	5 mg Q4H or 5mg IVB followed by an infusion at 1 mg/hr for 10 hours: maximum dose 30 mg (inpatients) and 15 mg (outpatients) in 24 hours	Onset: 10 min. Duration: 6–24 hours	
	Thiethylperazine maleate	Torecan®[f] Norzine®[g]	IM	10 mg QD-TID	—	Drowsiness, extrapyramidal side effects (dystonia, torticollis, akathisia, gait disturbances), hypotension
			PO	10 mg QD-TID	Onset: 30–60 min. Duration 3–4 hours	
			PR	10 mg QD-TID	Onset: 45–60 min.	
Corticosteroids	Dexamethasone	Decadron®[h]	IV	4–20 mg (10–20 mg given x 1, otherwise Q4–6H)	half life = 3–4 hours	Dyspepsia, hiccoughs, increased appetite, euphoria, insomnia, fluid retention, hyperglycemia
		Hexadrol®[i]	PO	4–8 mg Q4H x 4 doses	Peak 1–2 hours, Duration: 2 days	

(Continued on next page)

Table 16. Antiemetic Therapy: Select Pharmacologic Agents for the Control of Chemotherapy-Induced Nausea and Vomiting (Continued)

Classification	Generic Name	Trade Name(s)	Route	Dose/Schedule	Duration of Action	Adverse Events
Corticosteroids (cont.)	Prednisone		PO	2.5–15 mg Q4–12H	Peak 1–2 hours	Duration: 1–1.5 days	Dyspepsia, hiccoughs, increased appetite, euphoria, insomnia, fluid retention, hyperglycemia
Butyrophenones	Haloperidol	Haldol®[j]	IM PO IV	2–5 mg Q2H × 3–4 doses 2–5 mg Q2H × 3–4 doses 2 mg × 1	Onset: 15–30 min. Duration: 3–6 hours Onset: 40 min. Duration: 4–6 hours Onset: 15–30 min. Duration: 3–6 hours	Sedation, akathisia, extrapyramidal reactions, orthostatic hypotension
	Droperidol	Inapsine®[k]	IM IV	2–5 mg Q4–6H 2–5 mg Q4–6H or drip	Onset: 3–10 min. — Duration: 3–6 hours	Sedation, akathisia, extrapyramidal reactions, hypotension
Cannabinoids	Dronabinol	Marinol®[f]	PO	2.5–10 mg 1–3 hours before chemotherapy, then Q2H × 4–6 doses/day	— —	Sedation, dry mouth, euphoria or dysphoria, dizziness, orthostatic hypotension
Drugs used to augment antiemetics	Diphenhydramine	Benadryl®[l]	PO IM IV	25–50 mg Q4H PRN 25–50 mg Q4H PRN 25–50 mg Q4H PRN	Peak 1–3 hours. Duration: 4–7 hours Onset: 30 min. Duration: 4–7 hours Onset: Immediate. Duration: 4–7 hours	Sedation, dizziness, blurred vision/diplopia, dry mouth
	Lorazepam	Ativan®[m]	IV PO SL	1–2 mg/m², not exceeding 3 mg 0.5–2 mg 0.5–2 mg	Peak 1–3 hours. Duration: 4–8 hours — Duration 3–6 hours	Sedation, anterograde amnesia, dizziness, weakness, unsteadiness, disorientation, hypotension

[a] Glaxo Wellcome Oncology/HIV, Inc., Research Triangle Park, NC; [b] SmithKline Beecham Pharmaceuticals, Philadelphia, PA; [c] Hoechst Marion Roussel, Kansas City, MO; [d] A.H. Robins Company, Inc., Richmond, VA; [e] Schering Corporation, Kenilworth, NJ; [f] Roxane Laboratories, Inc., Columbus, OH; [g] The Purdue Frederick Company, Norwalk, CT; [h] Merck & Co., Inc., West Point, PA; [i] Organon Inc., West Orange, NJ; [j] McNeil Pharmaceutical, Raritan, NJ; [k] Janssen Pharmaceutica, Titusville, NJ; [l] Warner Wellcome, Morris Plains, NJ; [m] Wyeth-Ayerst Laboratories, Philadelphia, PA

Note. From "Serotonin Antagonists: State of the Art Management of Chemotherapy-Induced Emesis," by L.B. Cleri, 1995, *Oncology Nursing: Treatment and Support, 2*(1), pp. 1–19. Copyright 1995 by Lippincott-Raven. Adapted with permission.

(c) Methotrexate

(d) Cytosine arabinoside (Cytarabine®, Immunex Corp., Seattle, WA)

(e) Dactinomycin/actinomycin-D (Cosmegen®, Merck & Company, Inc., West Point, PA)

(f) Doxorubicin

(g) Azacitidine (5-azacytidine)

(h) Hydroxyurea (Hydea®, Bristol-Myers Squibb Oncology, Princeton, NJ)

(i) Nitrosoureas

b) Incidence

(1) Incidence varies with dose, drug, and administration schedule and is reported to be as high as 75% in patients receiving chemotherapy (Slichenmyer et al., 1993; Smith & Charmarro, 1978).

(2) Duration of diarrhea depends on the dose, drug, and administration schedule (Basch, 1987).

c) Assessment

(1) Risk factors

(a) Combination chemotherapy and radiation therapy to the pelvis that leads to additional cellular destruction of the bowel lumen

(b) Concurrent medications that cause diarrhea (e.g., corticosteroids, antibiotics) (Goodman & Riley, 1997)

(c) Neutropenic sepsis (e.g., *Clostridium difficile* or candidiasis) (Camp-Sorrell, 1997)

(d) Nutritional therapies (e.g., tube feedings, dietary supplements)

(e) Antiemetic therapy (e.g., metoclopramide)

(2) Physical exam

(a) Monitor bowel sounds, cramping, and distention.

(b) Assess for fecal impaction.

(3) Subjective measurement

(a) Assess the pattern of elimination in relation to treatments (i.e., onset, duration, frequency, consistency, amount).

(b) Assess dietary history, including intake of contributing factors (e.g., irritating foods, alcohol, coffee, fiber, fruit).

(4) Objective measurement

(a) Monitor intake and output.

(b) Monitor weight.

(c) Monitor laboratory data.

i) Stool cultures to rule out infectious causes

ii) Electrolyte balance, specifically potassium

d) Collaborative management

(1) Monitor number, amount, and consistency of bowel movements.

(2) Replace fluid and electrolytes, including potassium.

(3) Administer antidiarrheal medication to reduce stool frequency, volume, and peristalsis.

e) Patient education

(1) Instruct the patient about a low-residue, high-protein, high-calorie diet to provide bowel rest (e.g., applesauce, bananas, rice).

(2) Instruct the patient to eliminate from diet foods that are irritating to the bowel (e.g., alcohol, coffee, cold liquids, fresh fruits, popcorn, raw vegetables).

(3) Encourage the patient to drink six to eight glasses of water daily to restore fluid balance.

(4) Implement a liquid diet if diarrhea becomes severe. Serve food at room temperature. Hot and cold foods may aggravate diarrhea.

(5) Instruct the patient to avoid milk products and chocolate (including in cooking) in the event of a lactose intolerance.

(6) Instruct the patient about symptoms associated with hypokalemia, including weakness and fatigue.

(7) Advise patients with severe diarrhea to decrease activity. Bed rest will provide rest and decrease peristalsis.

(8) Advise the patient to clean rectal area with mild soap and water after each bowel movement to decrease the risk of infection and skin irritation.

Moisture-barrier ointment may provide additional protection.

(9) Instruct the patient to take warm sitz baths.

3. Mucositis

a) Pathophysiology (Beck, 1992): The epithelial cells of the oral mucosa are destroyed, causing an inflammatory response and denudation of the oral mucosa by the following mechanisms.

(1) Directly by the cytotoxic effects of chemotherapy drugs on the rapidly dividing epithelial cells of the oral mucosa

(2) Indirectly by bone marrow suppression

b) Incidence of overall oral complications

(1) Adult patients with leukemia: 23%–80% (Nieweg, Van Tinteren, Poelhuis, & Abraham-Inpijn, 1992)

(2) Adult patients with solid tumors: 40% (Nieweg et al., 1992)

(a) Carcinomas and sarcomas: 12%

(b) Lymphomas: 33%

c) Assessment

(1) Risk factors and specific populations at risk because of the occurrence of one or more of the following.

(a) Stomatotoxic antineoplastics: antitumor antibiotics, antimetabolites, alkylating agents (especially with high-dose continuous infusions) (Nieweg et al., 1992; Peterson & Schubert, 1992)

(b) Concurrent radiation, locally to head and neck, and total body irradiation

(c) Poor oral hygiene and gingival diseases (Beck, 1992; Peterson & Schubert, 1992)

(d) Elderly patients and those 20 years old or younger

i) Elderly patients are at risk because they tend to have decreased keratinization and salivary flow (Ofstehage & Magilvy, 1986).

ii) Children are at risk because they tend to have high mitotic activity, including their oral mucosa. They may have metal dental braces, which enhance microbial growth (Ofstehage & Magilvy, 1986).

(e) History of alcohol and/or tobacco use (Patients with head and neck cancer are at particular risk.) (Beck, 1992)

(f) Poor nutritional status

i) Dehydration causes altered mucosal integrity.

ii) Malnutrition (i.e., decreased protein-calorie intake) may cause altered mucosal integrity and decreased ability to heal (Beck, 1992).

(g) Patients with nasopharyngeal cancers

(h) Infiltration of leukocytes into the capillaries of oral cavity/gingiva in patients with leukemia

(i) Immunosuppression (i.e., patients undergoing BMT experience the indirect effects of pancytopenia and aplasia) (Dreizen, McCredie, Dicke, Zander, & Peters, 1979)

(j) Drugs or therapies that alter mucous membranes (e.g., antihistamines and oxygen therapy, which dry mucous membranes)

(k) History of herpes simplex virus seropositivity

(l) Renal or hepatic impairment

(2) Clinical manifestations

(a) Initial presenting symptoms of mucositis: burning sensation with no physical changes in oral mucosa, sensitivity to heat and cold, and sensitivity to salty and spicy foods and citrus juice (Nieweg et al., 1992). The incidence and severity of mucositis has decreased significantly with concomitant use of hematopoietic colony stimulating factors.

(b) Changes in taste and ability to swallow

(c) Pain upon swallowing or talking

(d) Edema of oral mucosa and tongue

(e) Mucosal ulcerations

(3) Physical examination

(a) Examine the lips, tongue, and oral mucosa for color, moisture, texture, and integrity (Beck, 1992).

(b) Assess for changes in taste, voice, ability to swallow, or comfort during swallowing (Beck, 1992).

(4) Assessment guides aid in evaluating and documenting changes in oral status (see Table 17).

d) Collaborative management

(1) Prevention

(a) Promote a well-balanced nutritional state, including a protein intake greater than 1 g/kg of body weight, adequate daily allowance of vitamins B and C, and a daily fluid intake of at least 2,000 ml.

(b) Encourage a diet that includes high-density and fibrous foods to cleanse the teeth and massage the gums and to avoid sugar-containing foods, which create a medium for bacterial growth, particularly if oral hygiene is irregular.

(c) Promote consistent, thorough oral hygiene by instructing the patient to brush, floss (only if previously part of regular oral hygiene), and rinse after each meal and before bedtime.

(d) Recommend a dental examination prior to instituting chemotherapy.

(2) Interventions

(a) Encourage the use of oral agents to promote cleansing, debridement, and comfort. Research has not determined the best solution; however, mouthwashes with more than

Table 17. Oral Assessment Guide					
	Tools for	**Methods of**	Numerical and Descriptive Ratings		
Category	**Assessment**	**Measurement**	**1**	**2**	**3**
Voice	Auditory	Converse with patient.	Normal	Deeper or raspy	Difficulty talking or painful
Swallow	Observation	Ask patient to swallow. To test gag reflex, gently place blade on back of tongue and depress.	Normal swallow	Some pain on swallowing	Unable to swallow
Lips	Visual/palpatory	Observe and feel tissue.	Smooth, pink, and moist	Dry or cracked	Ulcerated or bleeding
Tongue	Visual/palpatory	Feel and observe appearance of tissue.	Pink, moist, and papillae present	Coated or loss of papillae with a shiny appearance with or without redness	Blistered or cracked
Saliva	Tongue blade	Insert blade into mouth, touching the center of the tongue and the floor of the mouth.	Watery	Thick or ropy	Absent
Mucous membranes	Visual	Observe appearance of tissue.	Pink and moist	Reddened or coated (increased whiteness without ulcerations)	Ulcerations with or without bleeding
Gingiva	Tongue blade and visual	Gently press tissue with tip of blade.	Pink, stippled, and firm	Edematous with or without redness	Spontaneous bleeding or bleeding with pressure
Teeth or dentures (or denture-bearing area)	Visual	Observe appearance of teeth or denture-bearing area.	Clean and no debris	Plaque or debris in localized areas (between teeth if present)	Plaque or debris generalized along gum line or denture-bearing area

Note. Reprinted with permission of June Eilers, RN, MSN, CS, University of Nebraska Medical Center, Omaha, NE.

25% alcohol should be avoided because of irritation to the oral mucosa (see Table 18).

(b) Administer antifungal and antiviral agents prophylactically as ordered for patients likely to develop severe neutropenia. Prophylactic oral acyclovir (Zovirax®, Glaxo Wellcome Inc., Research Triangle Park, NC) is useful in preventing and/or minimizing herpes simplex, especially in BMT recipients.

(c) Recommend annual dental checkups.

(d) Administer pain medications.

(5) Patient education

(a) Instruct the patient that consistent, thorough oral hygiene is the best prevention and treatment for mucositis.

(b) Instruct the patient to avoid lemon glycerin swabs, which promote drying and irritation.

4. Anorexia

a) Pathophysiology

(1) Chemotherapy-related: Changes in taste and smell resulting from antineoplastics, antibiotics, or immunosuppressives can manifest as absent or altered taste and often lead to a decreased food intake

(a) Cells of taste buds have a rapid turnover rate.

(b) Chemotherapy changes the reproduction of taste buds.

(c) Certain drugs cause a metallic taste (e.g., methotrexate, cisplatin) (Twycross & Lack, 1986).

(2) Disease-related: Tumors can secrete substances such as cytokines, interleukin 1 (IL-1), and tumor necrosis factor (TNF), that circulate and affect various regulatory mechanisms for hunger, satiety, and metabolism (Beck & Tisdale, 1987).

(3) Anatomical changes: Dysphagia, obstruction, mucosal atrophy, and ulceration

(4) Concurrent renal or hepatic disease

(5) Increased metabolic rate leading to a cachectic state (Camp-Sorrell, 1997)

(6) Changes in activity level resulting in fatigue

(7) Early satiety

(8) Pain

b) Incidence: Varies with drugs, doses, administration schedule, tumor burden, side effects of treatment, and general physical state. Initial development of anorexia can be different from anorexia associated with end-stage disease.

c) Assessment

(1) Dietary history

(a) Ask the patient about the types of foods and beverages that he or she likes or dislikes.

(b) Assess the patient's daily nutritional intake and record the amount and types of food and beverage he or she consumes.

(c) Assess whether a change in food intake has affected the patient's mood or relationships with others.

(d) Assess frequency, degree, duration, and patterns of anorexia.

(e) Determine the patient's ability to prepare or obtain food.

(2) Physical examination

(a) Monitor the patient's height and weight and compare to usual (pretreatment) weight. Weight loss greater than 10% of IBW is a poor prognostic factor (Blackburn, Maini, Bistrian, Wade, & Tayek, 1987).

(b) Assess for fluid retention.

(c) Assess for indicators of dehydration or electrolyte imbalance, such as confusion and decreased urinary output.

(3) Laboratory results that may indicate anorexia include

(a) Total lymphocyte count of less than 1,200/mm

(b) Serum albumin of less than 3.5 gm/dl

Table 18. Oral Agents Used to Treat Mucositis

Indication	Agent	Dosage	Action
To promote cleanliness (Beck, 1992)	Baking soda and H_2O	½ tsp. baking soda with 4 oz water	Debride oral mucosa
	Soft toothbrush and dental floss	After each meal and before bed	Debride oral mucosa and remove plaque
	Saline solution	½ tsp. salt with 8 oz water	Debride oral mucosa
	Fluoride	1% sodium fluoride daily	Prevent dental caries related to radiation therapy to the head and neck
	Chlorhexidine	15 cc swish and spit twice a day	May decrease risk of oral infection
To promote moisturizing	Saline solution	½ tsp. salt with 8 oz water	Moisturize oral mucosa
	Sugar-free candy	As needed	Stimulate production of saliva
	MoiStir™ ªᵃ	Administer topically	Salivary supplement
	Pilocarpine (Salagen® ᵇ)	5 mg orally three times a day	Stimulate production of saliva in xerostomia related to radiation therapy to head and neck. Note: contraindicated in uncontrolled asthma, narrow angle glaucoma. Treat overdose with atropine 0.5–1.0 mg subcutaneous or IV.
To maintain integrity of oral mucosa	Allopurinol (Tsavaris, Caragiauris, & Kosmidis, 1988)	Administer topically	Unknown, but may decrease intensity of mucositis and provide comfort
	Sucralfate (Solomon, 1986)	1 tablet in 15 cc water to make slurry. Swish and swallow three times a day.	Unknown, but may involve the binding of sucralfate to damaged mucosal surface proteins, thus forming a protective coating
	Vitamin E and beta-carotene (Hogan, 1984).	Puncture capsule and apply directly on lesions (Fischer, Knobf, & Durivage, 1993)	Exert natural protective action on mucosal membranes in radiation mucositis
To promote comfort	Diclonine hydrochoride	5–10 ml swish and spit every three to four hrs. (Fischer et al., 1993)	Local anesthetic
Topical anesthetics	Viscous lidocaine (Katon, 1981)	5 cc swish and spit prior to meals or four times daily.	Local anesthetic; may cause numbing
	Zilactin®ᶜ (Rodu, Russell, & Ray, 1988)	Topical application to lesion(s) prn	Burns upon administration
Topical anti-inflammatory agents	Antacids	15 cc every two hours	Coat oral tissues
	Combinations of diphenhydramine hydrochloride elixir, viscous lidocaine, nystatin	15 cc four times a day, swish and swallow	Soothing, antifungal
Systemic analgesics	Aspirin	650 mg every four hours	Reduce inflammation
	Acetaminophen	650–1,000 mg every 4 hours	Provide systemic pain relief
	Opioids (e.g., MSO_4)	Varies according to drug used	Provide systemic pain relief for severe oral discomfort

ªKingswood Laboratories, Inc., Indianapolis, IN; ᵇMGI Pharmaceuticals, Inc., Minneapolis, MN; ᶜZila Pharmaceuticals, Inc., Phoenix, AZ

(c) Decreased transferrin (Albumin and transferrin are visceral proteins that are early indicators of low protein stores.) (Blackburn et al., 1987)

(d) Electrolyte imbalance or decreased nitrogen or calcium

d) Collaborative management

(1) Consult a dietician.

(2) High-calorie, high-protein dietary supplements may be indicated.

(3) Studies of high-dose megestrol acetate (Megace®, Bristol-Myers Squibb Oncology, Princeton, NJ) have demonstrated increased appetite and weight gain in patients who are anorexic or cachectic (Tchekmedyian, 1993).

(4) Enteral nutrition is indicated when the patient cannot meet caloric requirements by regular intake.

(5) Total parenteral nutrition (TPN) is indicated when gastrointestinal function is altered or absent (e.g., patient unable to absorb nutrients from the gut because of small bowel fistula or obstruction).

(a) Consists of glucose, amino acids, vitamins, minerals, trace elements, and lipids

(b) Costs 10–20 times more to deliver than enteral feedings

(c) Increases risk of infection because of glucose content of solution, which provides growth medium for bacteria

(6) Alert patient to community resources (e.g., Meals on Wheels) to assist with nutrition.

(7) Administer electrolyte and mineral replacement as indicated.

(8) Obtain a physician's order to administer appetite stimulants (e.g., megestrol acetate).

e) Patient education

(1) Instruct the patient to weigh himself or herself weekly using the same scale at the same time of day.

(2) Instruct the patient to eat small, frequent meals.

(3) Incorporate high-protein foods into the patient's diet to minimize weight loss and increase energy.

(4) Avoid foods that are filling and gas-forming (e.g., broccoli, cabbage, fruits, carbonated beverages).

(5) Prior to meals, avoid large quantities of liquids that may reduce the intake of solid foods.

(6) Eat slowly to allow the stomach to empty while eating.

(7) Medicate for pain or nausea to minimize discomfort, if indicated.

(8) Instruct the patient that wine or other alcoholic beverages before meals may stimulate appetite.

(9) Instruct the patient to avoid odors that could suppress appetite.

(10) Experiment with the temperature of foods, which may stimulate appetite.

(11) Plan daily food-preparation activities to conserve energy.

(12) Experiment with approaches to eating and food preparation (e.g., dining out, ordering take-out, preparing large quantities and freezing portions for later, purchasing frozen dinners).

(13) Report symptoms associated with anorexia to the healthcare team.

(14) Report physical changes that require symptom management. Fatigue, anemia, and mouth sores are specific physical problems that can cause poor appetite.

5. Constipation

a) Pathophysiology: Neurotoxic effects of chemotherapy can cause decreased peristalsis or paralytic ileus (e.g., vinca alkaloids such as vincristine, vinblastine [Velban®, Eli Lilly and Company, Indianapolis, IN], vinorelbine [Navelbine®, Glaxo Wellcome Oncology/HIV, Research Triangle Park, NC]) (O'Rourke et al., 1993; Portenoy, 1987, Weber et al., 1993).

b) Incidence
  (1) The frequency varies with doses, drugs, and administration schedules and is reported as high as 33% in patients receiving vincristine (Portenoy, 1987).
  (2) The duration of constipation depends on dose, drug, and administration schedule (Portenoy, 1987; Wrenn, 1989).
c) Assessment
  (1) Risk factors
    (a) Bowel obstruction secondary to tumor in the gastrointestinal tract
    (b) Decreased peristalsis caused by opioid administration
    (c) Decreased mobility
    (d) Fluid and electrolyte imbalance (e.g., dehydration)
    (e) Decreased or low dietary fiber intake
    (f) Advanced age (i.e., over age 65) (Blesch, 1988)
    (g) Hypercalcemia
    (h) Use of other medications
       i) Antidepressants
       ii) Diuretics
       iii) Iron preparations
       iv) Laxatives
       v) Calcium-containing antacids
       vi) Phenothiazines
       vii) Antiemetics (ondansetron HCl [Zofran®, Glaxo Wellcome Oncology/HIV, Research Triangle Park, NC] and granisetron HCl [Kytril®, SmithKline Beecham Pharmaceuticals, Philadelphia, PA])
  (2) Assess patterns of elimination, including the amount and frequency of elimination and the urge to defecate.
  (3) Assess the patient's usual dietary pattern, focusing on fluid and fiber intake.
  (4) Assess mobility and activity level.
  (5) Determine the patient's history of laxative and cathartic use, including amounts taken.
  (6) Conduct a physical exam that includes bowel sounds, distention, flatus, and presence of impaction.
d) Collaborative management
  (1) Administer cathartics as appropriate in accordance with an institutional prophylactic bowel regimen to facilitate bowel function.
  (2) Bowel-retraining regimen should include increased physical activity or passive exercise. This will promote the urge to defecate by helping to move the feces into the rectum.
  (3) Provide a quiet, private environment away from distractions.
  (4) Help the patient to maintain usual bowel habits during hospitalization.
e) Patient education
  (1) Encourage the patient to drink warm liquids to stimulate bowel movement.
  (2) Instruct the patient about dietary interventions that will minimize constipation, such as increased fiber in diet. Fiber will cause feces to pass through the intestines more rapidly and decrease the occurrence of fecal impaction. High-fiber foods include bran, popcorn, corn, raisins, dates, vegetables, fruits, and whole grains.
  (3) Encourage the patient to drink at least eight glasses of fluid daily unless medically contraindicated.
  (4) Encourage the patient to exercise regularly.
  (5) Help the patient to develop a regular bowel program, using stool softeners and bulk additives, if necessary, rather than harsh laxatives.
  (6) Instruct the patient in how to recognize complications associated with constipation, such as fecal impaction.
C. Alopecia
  1. Pathophysiology
    a) Cells responsible for hair growth have high mitotic and metabolic rates; 85%–90% of follicles on the scalp are in the anagen (growth) phase of the hair cycle

(DeSpain, 1992a; Fischer, Knobf, & Durivage, 1993).

b) Germination of normal hair root tissue averages 0.35 mm of shaft every 24 hours.

c) Hair damage is either to the shaft or to the root.

(1) Hair shaft damage results in partial atrophy or necrosis of the bulb, which causes constriction. Hair breaks off at that point, causing the patchy, thinner hair (Welch & Lewis, 1980).

(2) Root damage is associated with complete alopecia. Hair falls out spontaneously or is lost during combing or washing.

2. Incidence

a) Most chemotherapy drugs are associated with some degree of alopecia.

b) The degree of alopecia depends upon drug dose, serum half-life, the use of prolonged infusions, and the use of combination therapy (Fischer et al., 1993).

3. Assessment

a) Risk factors

(1) Drug administered

(2) High-dose chemotherapy

(3) Other medical conditions (e.g., hypothyroidism, aging)

(4) Nonchemotherapy medications (e.g., propanol hydrochloride [Inderal®, Wyeth-Ayerst Laboratories, Philadelphia, PA], heparin sodium, lithium carbonate, prednisone, vitamin A, androgen preparations)

(5) Self-care practices (e.g., pretreatment hair condition, nutritional status)

(6) Concomitant radiotherapy to head (local effect)

b) Clinical manifestations

(1) Degrees of alopecia

(a) Grade 0—No loss

(b) Grade 1—Mild hair loss

(c) Grade 2—Pronounced or total hair loss

(2) Expected time frame

(a) Hair loss begins approximately two weeks after administration of the drug.

(b) Regrowth may take three to five months after che-

motherapy is complete because the anagen phase of hair follicles lasts three months.

c) Scalp alopecia causes little physical morbidity but significant psychological morbidity (Baxley, Erdman, Henry, & Roof, 1984).

4. Collaborative management

a) Scalp hypothermia

(1) Theoretically, devices used to decrease circulation to the scalp (e.g., scalp tourniquets) can decrease the effectiveness of chemotherapy because of the sanctuary effect the device creates for circulating tumor cells (DeSpain, 1992b).

(2) Because of concerns regarding sanctuary sites and metastasis, scalp hypothermia is not recommended (DeSpain, 1992b; Witman, Cadman, & Chen, 1981).

(3) FDA pulled ice caps from the market in 1990.

b) Vitamin E is not effective (Martin-Jimenez, Diaz-Rubio, Larriba, & Sangro, 1986; Perez et al., 1986).

c) Patients can use wigs and other head coverings (e.g., American Cancer Society's "Look Good . . . Feel Better" national program).

d) Plan psychosocial interventions. Recognize that hair loss often is the only visible sign of cancer.

5. Patient education

a) Instruct the patient about the rationale and expected time frame of hair loss and regrowth.

b) Instruct the patient on gentle hair care, avoiding permanent waves, avoiding peroxide coloring, and minimizing use of electric rollers and curling irons until regrowth has been long enough to warrant two haircuts. While no research base exists, hair breakage may be minimized by avoiding chemical treatments.

c) Instruct the patient about emotional support strategies.

D. Fatigue

1. Pathophysiology

a) Definition: energy deficit related to disease, treatment, activity, rest, symptom perception, and functional status (Nail, 1997)

b) The cause of fatigue is unknown, but several etiologies of fatigue are theorized.

(1) Biochemical factors, with alterations in cardiopulmonary and neuromuscular status: Neurological impairments may be central in nature as a result of altered motivation, spinal cord transmission, and motor neurons or peripheral in nature as a result of impairments in peripheral nerves, the neuromuscular system, or fiber activation (MacVicar, Winningham, & Nickel, 1989; Piper, 1991; Sahlin, 1992; Winningham et al., 1994).

(2) Fatigue associated with surgery, chemotherapy, radiation therapy, biological response modifiers, and diagnostic tests (Brophy & Sharp, 1991; Greenberg, Sawicka, Eisenthal, & Ross, 1992; Irwin, 1987; Nail & King, 1987; Piper et al., 1998; Skalla & Lacasse, 1992)

(3) Altered nutritional status resulting from anorexia, cachexia, poor nutritional intake, and weight loss

(4) Altered activity, sleep, and rest

(5) Uncontrolled pain

(6) Psychosocial factors related to coping mechanisms, depression, anxiety, motivation, perceived social support, financial factors, and cultural beliefs (Nail & King, 1987; Piper, 1991; Piper et al., 1998)

(7) Biological characteristics (e.g., age, sex, genetics, allergies)

(8) Environmental factors (e.g., noise, temperature)

2. Incidence

a) Symptom with the highest incidence in patients with cancer (Winningham et al., 1994).

b) Reported by 59%–100% of patients undergoing cancer treatment (Blesch et al., 1991; Nail & King, 1987; Skalla & Lacasse, 1992).

3. Assessment

a) Assess the patient for risk factors, including poor nutrition, immobility, insomnia, stress, anemia, hypoxia, infection/fever, pain, and treatment with surgery, chemotherapy, radiation, and/or biological response modifiers.

b) Assess the impact on activities of daily living (ADL), and distinguish between acute and chronic fatigue (Piper et al., 1998; Skalla & Lacasse, 1992).

(1) Acute onset: intermittent symptoms that last less than one month

(2) Chronic: extreme, generalized weakness or lack of energy that lasts longer than one month

c) Assess coexisting medical conditions, including hypertension, diabetes, thyroid or metabolic disorders, electrolyte imbalances, infection, and menopause.

d) Assess for use or nonuse of medications that may contribute to symptoms, including vitamins, caffeine, alcohol, and recreational drugs.

e) Assess fatigue level (Winningham et al., 1994).

(1) Patient description using linear analog scale (0 = no fatigue to 10 = worst fatigue)

(2) Location, onset, and duration of fatigue

(3) Pattern of fatigue (i.e., intermittent versus constant)

(4) Enhancing and alleviating factors

(5) Associated factors (e.g., pain)

4. Collaborative management

a) Evaluate ADL and encourage the patient to balance exercise, rest, and energy-enhancing activities (Aistars, 1987; Winningham, 1992)

b) Collaborate with the physician and correct the potential causes of fatigue (e.g., dehydration, anemia, electrolyte imbalances, oxygenation).

c) Provide anticipatory guidance regarding symptoms to the patient and family. Develop an individualized care plan (Nail & King, 1987; Winningham, 1992).

(1) Assist the patient and family with reorganization of activi-

ties and work schedules, en-couraging them to decrease or eliminate low-priority activities.

(2) Evaluate medications that may contribute to fatigue and develop strategies to offset its effects (e.g., add caffeine with pain medications)

d) Obtain a nutritional consult as needed.

e) Obtain a rehabilitation and/or physical therapy consult, as needed.

f) Obtain a consult from a psychiatric nurse, social worker, psycho-oncologist, or psychiatrist, as needed.

5. Patient education

a) Instruct the patient and family on the causes and contributing factors of fatigue (Skalla & Lacasse, 1992).

b) Encourage the patient and family to set goals based on realistic abilities and limitations. Encourage the patient to ask for help with personal responsibilities as needed.

c) Encourage the patient to keep an activity/fatigue journal to identify patterns of energy and fatigue during the day.

d) Instruct the patient and family about strategies for dealing with and alleviating fatigue based on baseline functional status (Graydon, Bubela, Irvine, & Vincent, 1995; Mock et al., 1994; Winningham, 1991, 1992; Winningham et al., 1994).

(1) Encourage the patient to perform aerobic activities for 20–30 minutes three times a week.

(2) Encourage the patient to take short, frequent periods of rest.

(3) Encourage the patient to perform energy-enhancing activities such as meditation, yoga, visualization, listening to relaxation tapes, and relaxing with nature.

(4) Encourage the patient and family to prioritize activities and plan high-priority activities at times of increased energy.

(5) Encourage the patient to eat a nutritious diet, based on the food pyramid, and to limit caffeine and alcohol

(6) Encourage the patient to develop a routine sleeping pattern.

(7) Encourage the patient and family to maintain a moderate-temperature environment.

e) Instruct the patient to report changes in energy level to his or her healthcare provider (Skalla & Lacasse, 1992).

E. Cardiac toxicity

1. Pathophysiology

a) DNA intercalators: decreased contractility of heart leading to increased workload and hypertrophy related to direct insult of myofibrils

b) High-dose fluorouracil: coronary artery spasm leading to ischemia, possibly associated with myocardial infarction (Anand, 1994; Labianca, Beretta, Clerici, Fraschini, & Luporini, 1982; Pottage, Holt, Ludgate, & Langlands, 1978)

c) High-dose cyclophosphamide: Endothelial damage leading to myocardial necrosis (Mills & Roberts, 1979; Wujcik & Downs, 1992)

d) Paclitaxel: unknown

2. Acuity

a) Acute

(1) Occurs within 24 hours of drug administration

(2) Is self-limiting

(3) Electrocardiography (ECG) changes such as sinus tachycardia or arrhythmias have lead to cardiac decompensation and collapse (Kaszyk, 1986); however, development of transient changes usually is not an indication of therapy (Allen, 1992).

(4) Exception is acute changes associated with fluorouracil, which warrant immediate discontinuation of drug (Akhtar, Salim, & Bano, 1993)

b) Subacute

(1) Symptoms seen within four to five weeks following therapy

(2) Causes fibrinous pericarditis and myocardial dysfunction, which is diagnosed with a radionuclide cardiac scan (mul-

tiple gated acquisition [MUGA] scan) (Kaszyk, 1986)
(3) Usually reversible
(4) Chemotherapy may or may not be stopped, depending on the patient.
c) Chronic
(1) Seen with cumulative doses of cardiotoxic drugs that cause myocardial weakening (e.g., anthracyclines)
(2) Enhanced if radiation therapy has been given to left thorax
(3) Multiple characteristics (see Table 19)
(4) Cardiotoxic chemotherapy is stopped.
3. Incidence (Allen, 1992)
a) Acute and subacute toxicity occur infrequently.
b) Chronic toxicity is related to cumulative dose.
4. Assessment
a) Risk factors
(1) Cardiotoxic drugs (see Table 19)
(2) High-dose therapy
(3) Administration schedule: Higher doses over a shorter period increase cardiotoxicity (Allen, 1992).
(4) Thoracic irradiation to the lungs or mediastinum (Carlson, 1992)
(5) Age
(a) Children have an increased risk because of preexisting malnutrition, biological differences, metabolism, tissue sensitivity, and intensity of pediatric chemotherapy regimens (Carlson, 1992; Kaszyk, 1986).
(b) The elderly are at risk because of the inability of their bodies to self-repair as easily as when they were younger and because of preexisting cardiac disease (Carlson, 1992; Kaszyk, 1986; Von Hoff, Rozencwieg, Layard, Slavik, & Muggia, 1977).
(6) History of hypertension (Kaszyk, 1986)
(7) Preexisting cardiac disease (Kaszyk, 1986)
(8) Smoking, because of its asso-

ciation with cardiac changes (Kaszyk, 1986)
(9) Malnutrition, which may increase cardiotoxicity (Obama, Cangir, & van Eys, 1983)
b) Additional assessment
(1) Check the results of baseline cardiac studies (e.g., ejection fraction) before administering the drug.
(2) Observe for clinical manifestations of congestive heart failure (CHF) such as tachycardia, shortness of breath, nonproductive cough, neckvein distention, ankle edema, gallop rhythm, rales, hepatomegaly, and cardiomegaly.
(3) Assess the cumulative dose of the applicable drug (e.g., doxorubicin), and document it in patient records.
(4) Assess heart rate, rhythm, and regularity, including murmurs, split sounds, and extra sounds.
(5) Assess electrolytes (e.g., potassium, calcium), which can interfere with cardiac function when abnormal.
5. Collaborative management
a) Administer medications as prescribed to treat CHF and support cardiac output (e.g., diuretics, inotropic cardiac medications, vasodilators, oxygen).
b) In some settings, cardiac protective iron chelating agents such as ICRF-187 may be administered during or prior to the administration of the chemotherapeutic drug (Speyer et al., 1992). Dexrazoxane (Zinecard®, Pharmacia & Upjohn Co., Kalamazoo, MI) may be administered to prevent doxorubicin-induced cardiotoxicity in patients with metastatic breast cancer who have received greater than 300 mg/m² of doxorubicin (Pharmacia & Upjohn Inc., 1996).
c) Develop an activity or exercise plan.
d) Institute dietary modifications (e.g., a low-salt diet), as necessary, for CHF.
e) Instruct the patient to avoid tobacco and alcohol use because of their stimulative effect on cardiac muscle.

NOTES

_____

_____

_____

_____

f) Expect to discontinue or reduce the dose of the antineoplastic agent if the ejection fraction is less than 55%.

g) Monitor results of ECG performed at three months, six months, and one year post-therapy.

h) Monitor results of a MUGA scan completed every five years.

6. Patient education

a) Instruct the patient that cardiotoxicity is a possible side effect of the drug (e.g., anthracyclines, high-dose fluorouracil, high-dose cyclophosphamide [Cytoxan®, Bristol-Myers Squibb Oncology, Princeton, NJ])

b) Instruct the patient about signs and symptoms of CHF and when to report to a nurse or physician.

c) Instruct the patient that chronic cardiotoxicity usually is dose-related and possibly irreversible.

d) Instruct the patient and family about strategies they can use to manage symptoms at home.

F. Pulmonary toxicity

1. Pathophysiology

a) Lung tissue is sensitive to the toxic effects of chemotherapy,

Table 19. Cardiotoxic Drugs			
Drug	**Incidence**	**Characteristics**	**Comments**
DNA intercalators			
Doxorubicin	Total dose < 550 mg/m², incidence 0.1%–1.2% (Kaszyk, 1986; Von Hoff et al., 1979) Total dose > 550 mg/m², incidence rises exponentially (Von Hoff et al., 1979) Total dose 1,000 mg/m², incidence nearly 50% (Carlson, 1992; Von Hoff et al., 1979)	EKG changes; nonspecific ST-T wave changes; premature ventricular and atrial contraction; low voltage QRS changes and sinus tachycardia (Kaszyk, 1986); decreased ejection fraction; cardio-myopathy with symptoms of congestive heart failure (CHF) (Carlson, 1992)	Chronic effects seen with cumulative doses may result in CHF. Concomitant administration of other antineoplastics (e.g., cyclophosphamide) have been implicated as risk factors; however, the exact synergism is unclear (Burns, 1992).
Daunorubicin	Total dose < 600 mg/m², incidence 0%–41% (Kaszyk, 1986) Total dose 1,000 mg/m², incidence 12% (Kaszyk, 1986)		Chronic effects similar to doxorubicin, but higher cumulative doses may be tolerated (Von Hoff et al., 1977).
Dactinomycin	Incidence rare (Kaszyk, 1986)		Assessment complicated by concomitant combination chemotherapy (including anthracyclines) or prior mediastinal radiation.
Mitoxantrone	Total dose > 100 mg/m², with prior exposure to anthracyclines, transient EKG changes, incidence 28% (Kaszyk, 1986) Total dose > 160 mg/m², incidence 44% Without prior exposure to anthracyclines, incidence of decreased ejection fraction and CHF 2.1%–12.5% (Kaszyk, 1986; Von Hoff et al., 1977)		
High-dose therapy			
Cyclophosphamide	Not seen with cumulative doses or standard doses (Allen, 1992) Increased with high-dose therapy > 180–200 mg/kg/d x four days	Diminished QRS complex on EKG; cardiomegaly; pulmonary congestion (Gardner et al., 1993)	May result in acute lethal pericarditis and hemorrhagic myocardial necrosis (Mills & Roberts, 1979; Wujcik & Downs, 1992)
5-Fluorouracil	Incidence 1.6% (Labianca et al., 1982)	Angina, palpitations, sweating, and/or syncope (Akhtar et al., 1993)	May be treated prophylactically or therapeutically with long-acting nitrates or calcium channel blockers (Eskilsson, Albertsson, & Mercke, 1988)
Taxanes			
Paclitaxel	Incidence unknown	Asymptomatic bradycardia, hypotension, asymptomatic ventricular tachycardia, atypical chest pain	Toxicity has been documented as asymptomatic bradycardia (40–60 bpm), hypotension, asymptomatic ventricular tachycardia, and atypical chest pain. A baseline EKG, patient history, and cardiac assessment should be performed prior to treatment; however, routine cardiac monitoring during infusion is not recommended (Arbuck, Adams, & Strauss, 1992; Fischer et al., 1993; Rowinsky et al., 1991).

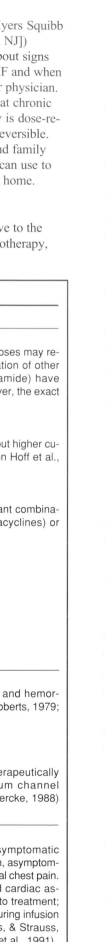

causing direct damage to the alveoli and capillary endothelium (Kriesman & Wolkove, 1992; Wickham, 1986).
  b) Most common types of pulmonary toxicity
    (1) Pulmonary edema (noncardiogenic): Acute onset related to capillary leak syndrome
    (2) Hypersensitivity pneumonitis
    (3) Pulmonary fibrosis and pneumonitis
      (a) Destruction to the alveolar/capillary endothelium, leading to changes in interstitial fibroblasts
      (b) Occurrence of delayed or abnormal tissue regeneration
2. Incidence
  a) Varies according to agent
  b) Difficult to determine at times because of combination therapies
  c) High incidence of pulmonary edema with interleukin-2 (often dose-limiting with high-dose therapy)
  d) Increased incidence with thoracic radiation therapy
3. Assessment
  a) Risk factors
    (1) Impaired drug excretion
      (a) Renal dysfunction may cause delayed drug excretion and increased pulmonary toxicity, especially with bleomycin.
      (b) Deteriorating creatinine clearance can be an important parameter in predicting pulmonary pneumonitis (Van Barneveld et al., 1984).
    (2) High oxygen concentrations can enhance the pulmonary toxicity of bleomycin (Ginsberg & Comis, 1984).
    (3) Concurrent chemotherapy (bleomycin, carmustine [BiCNU® Bristol-Myers Squibb Oncology, Princeton, NJ)], cyclophosphamide, doxorubicin) and radiation therapy have been associated with interstitial pulmonary pneumonitis (Wickham, 1986).
    (4) The risk of pulmonary toxicity increases significantly after age 70 (Wickham, 1986).

    (5) Underlying lung disease: Chronic obstructive pulmonary disease (COPD), asthma, bronchitis, and a history of smoking contribute to chemotherapy-induced pulmonary toxicity (Wickham, 1986).
  b) Clinical manifestations: Onset of hypersensitivity pneumonitis usually occurs 7–10 days after administration. Pulmonary fibrosis can be an acute or chronic reaction.
  c) Physical assessment
    (1) Percuss and auscultate the lungs. Assess location and degree of adventitious breath sounds (e.g., rales, rhonchi, wheezes).
    (2) Assess depth, rhythm, and effort of respiratory breathing.
    (3) Note chest symmetry and retraction of intercostal muscles.
    (4) Note accessory muscle use.
    (5) Determine the presence of a cough and the amount, color, and productive nature of sputum.
    (6) Note skin and mucous membrane color (dusky, ashen, or cyanotic color).
    (7) Monitor the results of pulse oximetry and arterial blood gases.
    (8) Obtain a chest x-ray.
    (9) Monitor pulmonary function tests.
4. Collaborative management
  a) Hold chemotherapy and notify a physician.
  b) Initiate fluid restriction if pulmonary edema is problematic.
  c) Administer corticosteroids and antibiotics as ordered.
  d) Provide supportive therapy (e.g., vasopressors, diuretics, artificial ventilation) for acute episodes.
  e) Provide oxygen therapy.
  f) Follow-up recommendations
    (1) Monitor pulmonary function tests as indicated.
    (2) Obtain a chest x-ray.
5. Patient education
  a) Provide patient education regarding symptoms associated with pulmonary toxicity (e.g., dyspnea, chest pain, shallow breathing, chest wall discomfort).

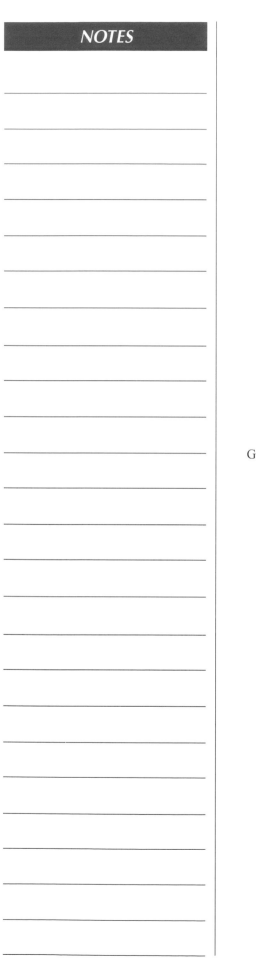
b) Teach the patient that raising the head of the bed may facilitate breathing.

c) Instruct the patient to conserve energy by performing daily activities when his or her energy level is highest.

d) Teach the patient and family methods to decrease symptoms of dyspnea by exercising to tolerance, practicing pursed-lip breathing, refraining from smoking, and using a small fan.

e) Teach the patient to take an opioid (usually morphine) as prescribed by his or her physician because opioids may relieve the discomfort caused by air hunger.

f) If at risk for pulmonary edema, teach the patient to restrict fluid.

g) Review the safety issues related to oxygen administration (e.g., flammable potential).

h) Explore with the patient his or her wishes regarding intubation and resuscitation status to establish advance directives.

G. Hemorrhagic cystitis

1. Pathophysiology: bladder mucosal irritation and inflammation resulting from contact with acrolein, the metabolic by-product of cyclophosphamide and ifosfamide (Ifex®, Bristol-Myers Squibb Oncology, Princeton, NJ).

2. Incidence

   a) Cyclophosphamide—intermittent or chronic low-dose cyclophosphamide (less than 1,000 mg): 10% (Patterson & Reams, 1992)

   b) High-dose cyclophosphamide for BMT (at least 120 mg/kg)—40% (Patterson & Reams, 1992)

   c) Ifosfamide—29% frank hematuria; combined incidence of microscopic and gross hematuria approaches 50%.

3. Assessment

   a) Risk factors

     (1) Cyclophosphamide administered intravenously may result in a greater risk for toxicity than when administered orally. Toxicity may occur with a single dose of IV cyclophosphamide or with up to 57 mg/kg administered over two years (Stillwell & Benson, 1988).

     (2) Pediatric populations may be at an increased risk with lower single and total doses of cyclophosphamide. Exact etiology is unclear, but it may result from the rate of administration versus age (Stillwell & Benson, 1988).

     (3) Prior radiation therapy to the pelvis or bladder increases the risk of hemorrhagic cystitis (Stillwell & Benson, 1988).

   b) Clinical manifestations

     (1) Dysuria, frequency, and burning upon urination

     (2) Blood in urine

4. Collaborative management

   a) Preventing hemorrhagic cystitis

     (1) Assess BUN, creatinine, routine urinalysis, and urine culture as needed to rule out renal pathology and urinary tract infection.

     (2) Instruct adult patients to increase their oral fluid intake (three liters/day). Provide vigorous IV hydration if they are unable to drink and retain fluid.

     (3) Encourage frequent voiding, including throughout the night as necessary.

     (4) Administer a prophylactic chemoprotectant (e.g., mesna [Mesnex®, Bristol-Myers Squibb Oncology, Princeton, NJ]) when administering high-dose cyclophosphamide and any dose of ifosfamide. Mesna binds to acrolein in the bladder, inactivating it. The inactive compound then is flushed out of the bladder.

       (a) Examples of a mesna dose

         i) For ifosfamide: Administer mesna at 20%–39% of the ifosfamide dose (Dorr, 1991) 15 minutes before and four and eight hours after ifosfamide (Zalupski & Baker, 1988). It is also administered as a continuous infusion at 100% of the ifosfamide dose preceded by a loading dose of mesna (Fischer et al., 1993).

         ii) For high-dose cyclophosphamide: Administer mensa at 60%–120% of the cyclophosphamide dose 15 minutes before and four and eight hours after the cyclophosphamide dose (Shepherd et al., 1991).

b) Managing hemorrhagic cystitis
(1) Stop drug administration if evidence of gross hematuria or cystitis is noted.
(2) Place a three-way Foley catheter for continuous irrigation with saline or acetylcysteine (Mucomyst®, Bristol-Myers Squibb, Princeton, NJ) to bathe the bladder and decrease clotting (Patterson & Reams, 1992).
(3) Administer aminocaproic acid (Amicar®, Immunex Corporation, Seattle, WA) intravenously or orally, if indicated, to promote clotting.
(4) Electrocautery or cryosurgery may be used if bleeding is not controlled with irrigations or aminocaproic acid (Wujcik & Downs, 1992).
(5) As a last resort, cystectomy may be necessary for severe hemorrhagic cystitis.

c) Follow-up recommendations
(1) Annual urinalysis, urine cytology, and cystoscopy (Stillwell & Benson, 1988)
(2) Excretory urograms periodically for patients with gross hematuria, new microhematuria, or abnormal urine cytologic findings or persistent irritative voiding symptoms (Stillwell & Benson, 1988)

5. Patient education
a) Instruct the patient that hemorrhagic cystitis is a possible side effect of cyclophosphamide or ifosfamide therapy.
b) Instruct the patient to report signs and symptoms of hemorrhagic cystitis.
c) Encourage the patient receiving oral cyclophosphamide therapy to void frequently and to take medication as early in the day as possible.
d) Instruct the patient to drink six to eight glasses of fluid daily, to empty bladder every four to six hours, and to notify nurse or physician if unable to do so.

H. Hepatotoxicity
1. Pathophysiology: Caused by a direct toxic effect to the liver when drugs are metabolized. Effects include fatty changes, hepatocellular necrosis, cholestasis, hepatic fibrosis, and parenchymal cell damage (McDonald & Tirumali, 1984).
2. Incidence: See Table 20.
3. Assessment
a) Risk factors
(1) Prior liver infection or damage (e.g., hepatitis, cirrhosis)
(2) Hepatotoxic drugs (present an increased risk with higher doses)
(3) Diabetes mellitus
(4) Prior tumor involvement of the liver
(5) Prior irradiation of the liver
(6) History of alcoholism, especially with cirrhosis
(7) Concurrent administration of hepatotoxic drugs
(8) Advancing age resulting in declining liver function
(9) Total bilirubin greater than 2 mg/100 dl
b) Clinical manifestations
(1) Jaundice
(2) Ascites
(3) Fatigue
(4) Anorexia
(5) Nausea
(6) Hyperpigmentation of the skin
(7) Right upper-quadrant pain
(8) Hepatomegaly
(9) Changes in urine or stool color
c) Assess liver function tests, obtain baseline prior to beginning therapy, and monitor consecutive levels.
4. Collaborative management
a) Avoid other hepatotoxic drugs if liver function test results are abnormal.
b) Chemotherapy may be reduced based on elevated liver function studies. However, with the exception of doxorubicin, this practice is controversial because of the paucity of protective studies validating it (Perry, 1992)
c) Follow-up recommendations
(1) Periodic evaluation of liver function tests
(2) Physical exam, abdominal ul-

Table 20. Hepatotoxicity

Classification	Incidence	Comments
Alkylating agents		
Cyclophosphamide	Rare	Exception is > 3 grams used in bone marrow transplant (Perry, 1992).
Nitrosoureas		
Carmustine	26% at low doses	Usually not clinically significant (DeVita et al., 1965); however, may be associated with severe veno-occlusive disease when used during bone marrow transplant (McDonald, Hinds, Fisher, & Schoch, 1993).
Lomustine	26% (Hoogstraten et al., 1973)	
Streptozocin	15%–67% (Broder & Carter, 1973)	
Antimetabolites		
Methotrexate	24% with oral administration	Cumulative dose important in degree of hepatotoxicity (Podurgiel, McGill, Luwig, Taylor, & Muller, 1973).
6-Mercaptopurine	Unknown	Seen only when doses exceed 2 mg/kg/d (Einhorn & Davidson, 1964).
Cytosine arabinoside	Unknown	Incidence difficult to establish because patient population receives treatment that confounds variables (e.g., patients receive frequent blood transfusions which could cause liver alterations). Patients on cytosine arabinoside are poor candidates for liver biopsy, and cause of hepatotoxicity cannot be established (Perry, 1992).
5-Fluorouracil	Rare (Perry, 1992)	
Antitumor antibiotics		
Doxorubicin	Rare (Perry, 1992)	May be lower than other anthracyclines (Shenkenberg & Von Hoff, 1986).
Mitoxantrone	Rare	
Bleomycin	Rare (Blum, Carter, & Agre, 1973)	
Mitomycin	Unknown (Perry, 1992)	
Plicamycin	16% (Green & Donehower, 1984)	
Plant alkaloids		
Vincristine	Rare (Perry, 1992)	
Etoposide	Rare	Not seen at standard doses; higher doses may cause reversible liver enzyme changes (Johnson, Greco, & Wolff, 1983).
Paclitaxel	7%–22% (Mead Johnson Oncology Products, 1994)	
Miscellaneous agents		
Cisplatin	Rare	Rare at standard dose, but may be increased with higher doses (Cavalli, Tschopp, Sonntag, & Zimmerman, 1978; Pollera, Ameglio, Nardi, Vitelli, & Marolla, 1987).
Carboplatin	Unknown (Perry, 1992)	
L-asparaginase	42%–87% (Capizzi, Bertino, & Handschumacher, 1970)	
Hydroxyurea	Rare (Thurman et al., 1963)	
Amsacrine	Unknown (Arlin et al., 1980)	
Dacarbazine	Unknown (Ceci et al., 1988)	

trasound, or abdominal CT for chronic abnormalities in liver function tests to establish etiology

5. Patient education
   a) Instruct the patient to avoid alcoholic beverages if hepatotoxicity is noted.
   b) Instruct the patient that hepatotoxicity is a possible side effect of selected chemotherapy agents.
   c) Instruct the patient about the signs and symptoms of liver failure (e.g., jaundice, liver tenderness, changes in urine or stool color).

I. Nephrotoxicity
   1. Pathophysiology (Lydon, 1980)
      a) Direct cell damage to the glomerulus, renal blood vessels, and/or different parts of the nephron
      b) Precipitation of metabolites in the acid environment of the urine that causes obstructive nephropathy
   2. Incidence: See Table 21.
   3. Assessment
      a) Risk factors
         (1) Advancing age, during which the kidneys become slightly smaller and renal function decreases (Patterson & Reams, 1992)
         (2) Directly by preexisting renal disease or indirectly by connective, liver, or cardiac disease (Patterson & Reams, 1992)
         (3) Poor nutritional status
         (4) Hypovolemia, which may increase the risk of acute renal failure (Jenkins & Rieselbach, 1982)
         (5) Administration of other nephrotoxic drugs (e.g., NSAIDs, aminoglycoside antibiotics, amphotericin-B, cyclosporine) (Raymond, 1984)
         (6) Extravascular fluid shifts
      b) Clinical manifestations (Patterson & Reams, 1992)
         (1) Increasing serum creatinine
         (2) Declining creatinine clearance
         (3) Hypomagnesemia
         (4) Proteinuria
         (5) Hematuria
      c) Laboratory values (Lydon, 1986)
         (1) BUN
            (a) Assess baseline and consecutive levels.
            (b) Roughly estimate renal function (very sensitive to hydration status and elevated in presence of dehydration).
            (c) Usually hold the chemotherapy agent for serum BUN value of greater than 22 mg/dl.
         (2) Serum creatinine
            (a) Assess baseline and consecutive levels.
            (b) A specific and sensitive indicator of renal function
            (c) Usually hold the chemotherapy agent for serum

Table 21. Nephrotoxicity

Drug	Incidence	Comments
Cisplatin	25%–30%	May cause acute tubular injury following single-dose 50 mg/m² IV (Evans, 1991; Lydon, 1986)
Mitomycin-C	2%–10%	May cause drug-associated hemolytic uremic syndrome with cumulative doses greater than 60 mg (Hrozencik & Connaughton, 1988; Vogelzang, 1991)
Streptozocin	Variable	May cause tubular interstitial nephritis and tubular atrophy (Myerowitz, Sartiano, & Cavallo, 1976). However, nephrotoxicity is rarely reported with doses of 1–1.5 g/m²/week (Sadoff, 1979; Vogelzang, 1991).
Carmustine/lomustine	Common with cumulative doses > 1,500 mg/m² (Lydon, 1986; Patterson & Reams, 1992)	Interstitial fibrosis and glomerular sclerosis (Vogelzang, 1991); renal toxicity onset is late, occuring months to years after chemotherapy (Patterson & Reams, 1992).
Methotrexate	10% with high-dose therapy	Prevented by concomitant hydration and urinary alkalinization. Tubular injury is precipitated by methotrexate entering renal tubules during high-dose therapy or acidic urine pH (Lydon, 1986; Vogelzang, 1991).
Ifosfamide	Less than 10%	Incidence may increase with existing renal dysfunction or prior cisplatin therapy (Vogelzang, 1991).

creatinine value of greater than 2 mg/dl.

(3) 12-hour creatinine clearance

(a) Assess baseline and consecutive levels.

(b) Creatinine clearance can be the most sensitive test for renal function (12-hour is as effective as 24-hour test and less costly).

(c) Accuracy is dependent on collecting all urine in a specified time.

(d) Usually hold chemotherapy agent for creatinine clearance value of less than 60 ml/min. or according to protocol/guideline.

(4) Urine cytology

(a) Assess changes in urine cytology (e.g., RBC, WBC, epithelial cells).

(b) Assess tubular damage.

(c) Very inaccurate in patients who are cachectic.

(5) Urine protein: Proteinuria indicates damage to the glomerular and tubular systems.

(6) Urine-specific gravity and osmolality

(a) Measures the kidneys' ability to concentrate or dilute urine

(b) Indicates the presence or absence of tubular and/or medullary damage

(7) Urine pH

(a) Measures the free hydrogen ion concentration in the urine

(b) Expresses the strength of the urine as a dilute acid of a base solution

(8) Serum electrolytes, especially magnesium and potassium levels

(a) Measure when giving high-dose chemotherapy, especially cisplatin.

(b) Assess for fluid imbalance.

d) Objective data

(1) Intake and output

(2) Weight

(3) Presence of edema

4. Collaborative management

a) Monitor renal function tests.

b) Institute hydration of 3,000 ml/day to prevent or minimize renal damage, especially with cisplatin and methotrexate.

c) Induce diuresis with either mannitol or furosemide when administering cisplatin (Evans, 1991)

d) Administer allopurinol to decrease uric acid production from high tumor-cell kill (e.g., acute leukemia, lymphoma, small-cell lung cancer, BMT). Discontinue allopurinol when peripheral WBC count falls to $1,000/mm^3$ or less.

e) Stop drug if creatinine does not return to baseline or if the patient develops proteinuria when receiving streptozocin (Zanosar®, Pharmacia and Upjohn Co., Kalamazoo, MI).

f) Prevent renal damage from high-dose methotrexate (greater than $100 mg/m^2$).

(1) Maintain alkylinization of urine with sodium bicarbonate to a pH level greater than 8.

(2) Administer leucovorin rescue within the recommended time frame.

(3) Avoid vitamin C, aspirin, NSAIDs, penicillins, and sulfa drugs 48 hours before and after methotrexate.

(4) Reduce subsequent doses based on degree of toxicity.

g) Follow-up recommendations

(1) Conduct periodic evaluations, including urinalysis, creatinine clearance, and serum chemistries.

(2) Declining renal function requires referral to nephrologist to assess damage and possibly provide further work-up and treatment.

5. Patient education

a) Instruct the patient that nephrotoxicity is a possible side effect of selected chemotherapy agents.

b) Reinforce the importance of patient compliance with preventive measures for nephrotoxicity.

(1) Accurately obtaining 12–24 hour urine for creatinine clearance

(2) Increasing fluid intake

(3) Complying with instructions to alkalinize urine, complete leucovorin rescue and/or allopurinol therapy, and avoid

use of drugs that potentiate renal dysfunction in combination with methotrexate (see Section *f)*, (1)–(3), page 82).

J. Neurotoxicity
1. Pathophysiology
   a) Direct chemotherapy toxicity on the nervous system
   b) Metabolic encephalopathy
   c) Intracranial hemorrhage or infection related to chemotherapy-induced coagulopathy or myelosuppression
2. Incidence: Exact incidence is unknown, but incidence is increasing with greater use of high-dose chemotherapy.
3. Assessment
   a) Risk factors
      (1) Regimens including high-dose methotrexate, high-dose cytosine arabinoside, vinblastine, vinorelbine, ifosfamide, vincristine, vindesine (Eldisine®, Eli Lilly and Company, Indianapolis, IN), cisplatin, or 5-fluorouracil
      (2) Administration of chemotherapy agents that cross the blood-brain barrier (e.g., high-dose methotrexate, cytosine arabinoside, nitrosoureas)
      (3) Intracarotid or intrathecal chemotherapy
      (4) Concomitant cranial radiotherapy
      (5) Age
         (a) Cerebellar neurotoxicity of cytosine arabinoside increases with increasing age. However, cytosine arabinoside neurotoxicity occurs only with high-dose therapy (greater than 100 mg/ml individual doses (Macdonald, 1991).
         (b) Children are at higher risk for ototoxicity because their inner ears are not fully developed.
      (6) Cumulative doses of vinca alkaloids, especially vincristine and taxanes (e.g., paclitaxel), induce peripheral neuropathies. Toxicity also occurs with high-dose therapy (e.g., greater then 60 g/m² of cisplatin), especially if renal function is poor.
      (7) Impaired renal function
      (8) Concurrent or subsequent administration of diuretics or aminoglycoside antibiotics may increase cisplatin-induced sensory neuropathy and ototoxicity and may increase cerebellar damage as a result of cytarabine administration (Hydzik, 1990).
4. Collaborative management
   a) Use assessment guidelines for early detection and treatment. Reduce drug dose or discontinue drug as ordered when neurological deficits are noted (e.g., fine motor losses, numbness, tingling, gait disturbances, constipation, change in mentation).
   b) Some reports have indicated that rapid administration of cisplatin increases risks of neurotoxicity; however, this conclusion is controversial (Hydzik, 1990) (see Table 22).
   c) Follow-up recommendations
      (1) Assess objective and subjective toxicities and subsequent functional impairment.
      (2) Consider consultation with a neurologist, a pain-management service, and a physical therapist.
5. Patient education
   a) Instruct the patient that neurotoxicity is a possible side effect of selected chemotherapy agents.
   b) Instruct the patient and family about the signs and symptoms of neurotoxicity and the importance of notifying the physician if they occur.

K. Sexual and reproductive dysfunction
1. Pathophysiology
   a) Definition
      (1) Impaired sexual and reproductive capacity caused by the biological process of cancer, the effects of treatment, and the psychological issues (Krebs, 1993).
      (2) Infertility occurs in men primarily through depletion of the germinal epithelium that lines the seminiferous tubules. Clinically, as testicular volume decreases, oligospermia or azoospermia occurs, resulting in infertility (Krebs, 1993).

Table 22. Neurotoxicity

Area of Neurological Deficit	Chemotherapeutic Agent	Assessment	Collaborative Management
Cerebrum Mental status	L-asparaginase Cisplatin Carboplatin Ifosfamide Pentostatin	Assess for confusion, memory loss, level of consciousness, seizures.	1. Use positive support and encouragement when assisting with activity. 2. Keep a consistent schedule for patients with memory loss to avoid frustration.
Peripheral nerves Sensory	Cisplatin Carboplatin Cytarabine Etoposide Paclitaxel Docetaxel Vinblastine Vincristine	Assess for decreased or absent deep tendon reflexes, numbness, decreased sensation, jaw pain, paresthesia of hands and feet.	1. Avoid extreme temperatures. 2. Use assistive devices as needed (e.g., instruments with large handles). 3. Medicate with opioids, antidepressants, and anticonvulsants for neuropathic pain (American Pain Society, 1992).
Motor	Paclitaxel Docetaxel Vinblastine Vincristine	Assess for foot drop, muscle weakness.	1. Exercise limbs by flexing and stretching four times daily. Use passive range of motion when patient is unable to assist (Dodd, 1991). 2. Use assistive devices (e.g., splints, braces, canes) with weakness and gait difficulty.
Autonomic nervous system	Vinblastine Vincristine	Assess for abdominal pain, constipation/ileus, bladder incontinence/atony.	1. Recommend a diet high in fiber. 2. Encourage adequate fluid intake (3,000 cc/day). 3. Administer laxatives and bowel stimulants as needed (Tenenbaum, 1989). 4. Begin a bowel program one-half hour after meals when gastrocolic reflex is strongest (Kelly & Mahon, 1988). 5. Instruct patient to follow a fluid and urination schedule with bladder incontinence. 6. Monitor for bladder infection related to urinary retention (Wahlquist, 1985).
Cerebellum	Cytarabine	Assess for ataxic tremor, loss of coordination, horizontal nystagmus, diplopia.	1. Discontinue drug as ordered when nystagmus occurs with other neurotoxicity (Barnett et al., 1985; Conrad, 1986). 2. Apply alternating eye patches every four hours to control diplopia. 3. Encourage patient to speak slowly and use short phrases with dysarthria. 4. Use alphabet boards and note pads to facilitate communication. 5. Institute safety precautions to prevent falls or bumping into objects. 6. Assist with ambulation, and use assistive devices as needed (Meehan & Johnson, 1992).
Meninges	Vincristine	Assess for meningismus, paralysis, loss of vision.	1. Turn patient every two hours to maintain skin integrity with paralysis.
Cranial nerves Olfactory		Assess for loss of smell.	
Optic	Cisplatin Carboplatin	Assess for papilledema, loss of vision using a Snellen chart.	1. Ambulate with assistance when visually impaired. 2. Orient patient to surroundings by touch, and keep surroundings consistent.
Oculomotor, trochlear, abducens	Cisplatin Carboplatin Cyclophosphamide	Assess for diplopia, nystagmus, alteration in color vision, papilledema.	See cerebellar management.
Trigeminal	Vincristine	Assess for jaw pain.	1. Medicate as needed for neuropathic jaw pain. 2. Provide a soft diet to minimize painful mastication.

(Continued on next page)

(3) Women experience sexual and reproductive dysfunction as a result of hormonal alterations or direct effects that cause ovarian fibrosis and follicular destruction. Follicle stimulating hormone (FSH) and luteinizing hormone (LH) levels are elevated and estradiol is decreased, leading to amenorrhea, menopausal symptoms, dyspareunia, and vaginal atrophy and dryness (Barton-Burke et al., 1996; Schilsky, Lewis, & Sherins, 1980).

b) Multiple causes for sexual and reproductive dysfunction exist.
  (1) Chemotherapy compromises fertility by exerting cytotoxic effects on gametogenesis. The degree of general effect is governed by the therapeutic regimen (type, dose, schedule) and duration of treatment (Sweet, Servy, & Karow, 1996).
  (2) Sexual dysfunction can be caused by the physical side effects of cancer treatments.
    (a) Pain
    (b) Nausea
    (c) Vomiting
    (d) Diarrhea
    (e) Weakness
    (f) Fatigue
    (g) Alopecia
    (h) Altered body image

  (i) Muscle atrophy
  (j) Neurologic changes
(3) Cancer and its treatment may result in psychological states that affect sexual desire (Dow, 1995; Dudas, 1993).
    (a) Anxiety
    (b) Depression
    (c) Dependency
    (d) Anger
2. Incidence
  a) Sexual dysfunction
    (1) Between 40%–l00% of patients report some evidence of sexual dysfunction following treatment (Derogatis & Kourlesis, 1981).
    (2) Sexual dysfunction frequently is underreported because it is not assessed by medical personnel.
    (3) The majority of male patients who receive antiandrogen therapy experience a major reduction in sex drive and are unable to attain or maintain an erection (Rousseau, Dupont, Labrie, & Couture, 1988).
  b) Reproductive dysfunction
    (1) Varies according to the agent and dose (e.g., more than 9 g of cyclophosphamide produces azoospermia) (Fairley, Barrie, & Johnson, 1972).
    (2) In women
      (a) A permanent cessation in menses increases nearer to age 40.

Table 22. Neurotoxicity (Continued)

Area of Neurological Deficit	Chemotherapeutic Agent	Assessment	Collaborative Management
Cranial nerves (cont.)			
Facial	Carboplatin Cisplatin Vincristine	Assess for facial palsies, alteration in taste.	See glossopharyngeal management.
Auditory	Cisplatin Prednisone	Assess for tinnitus, hearing loss using the Weber test and Rinne test, nystagmus, vertigo.	1. Report auditory changes reported by the patient. 2. Reduce or discontinue chemotherapy dose as ordered.
Glossopharyngeal	Cyclophosphamide Levamisole	Assess for dysphagia, taste alterations.	1. Assess food preferences and offer additional seasoning to improve taste and aroma (Dodd, 1991).
Vagus		Assess for hoarseness, dysphagia, dysphonia.	1. Encourage a soft diet with consistent texture for dysphagia. 2. Encourage patient to rest voice with hoarseness.

Note. From "The Neurotoxicity of Antineoplastic Agents," by J.L. Meehan and B.L. Johnson, 1992, *Current Issues in Cancer Nursing Practice Updates*, *1*(8), pp. 2–9. Copyright 1992 by J.B. Lippincott Co. Adapted with permission.

(b) Women younger than age 35 can tolerate much higher doses of chemotherapy without resultant infertility.

(c) Eighty percent of women under age 25 continue normal menses.

(3) Treatment with alkylating agents results in irreversible azoospermia in 80%–90% of men with Hodgkin's disease (Jaffe et al., 1988; Selby et al., 1988).

3. Assessment

a) Risk factors

(1) Treatment with specific chemotherapy agents (see Table 23)

(2) Concurrent medication such as sedatives, antihypertensives, and narcotics (see Table 24)

(3) Age

(4) Prior surgical procedures

(5) History of radiation therapy to the pelvis

(6) Hormonal therapy

(7) Fatigue

(8) Depression and/or other psychosocial stressors

(9) Chronic diseases (e.g., diabetes)

b) Clinical manifestations

(1) Sexual dysfunction

(a) Females

i) Decreased libido

ii) Dyspareunia

(b) Males

i) Decreased libido

ii) Mild, intermediate, or severe erectile dysfunction

iii) Difficulty maintaining an erection

iv) Premature ejaculation

Table 23. Chemotherapeutic Agents That Affect Sexual or Reproductive Function

Agent	Complication
Alkylating agents Busulfan Chlorambucil Cyclophosphamide Melphalan Nitrogen mustard	Amenorrhea, oligospermia, azoospermia, decreased libido, ovarian dysfunction, erectile dysfunction
Antimetabolites Cytosine arabinoside 5-Fluorouracil Methotrexate	No ovarian dysfunction as single agents; may potentiate dysfunction when combined with alkylating agents
Antitumor antibiotics Doxorubicin Plicamycin Dactinomycin	No ovarian dysfunction as single agents; may potentiate dysfunction when combined with alkylating agents
Plant alkaloids Vincristine Vinblastine	Retrograde ejaculation, erectile dysfunction Decreased libido, ovarian dysfunction, erectile dysfunction
Miscellaneous agents Procarbazine Androgens Antiandrogens Estrogens Antiestrogens Progestins Aminoglutethamide Corticosteroids Interferons	As with alkylating agents Masculinization in women Gynecomastia, impotence Gynecomastia, acne Irregular menses Menstrual abnormalities, libido changes Masculinization in women Irregular menses, acne Transient impotence

Note. From "Sexual and Reproductive Dysfunction," by L. Krebs, in S.L. Groenwald, M.H. Frogge, M. Goodman, and C.H. Yarbro (Eds.), *Cancer Nursing: Principles and Practice* (3rd ed.), p. 705, Boston: Jones & Bartlett. Copyright 1993 by Jones & Bartlett. Adapted with permission.

---

v) Difficulty reaching orgasm
(2) Reproductive dysfunction
  (a) Females
    i) Temporary or permanent amenorrhea
    ii) Early menopause and accompanying symptoms
    iii) Fertility may be impaired (follicular damage), but some ova are spared, accounting for irregular menses and/or delayed recovery of menstrual function.
    iv) Ovarian fibrosis and sterility
    v) Abnormal hormone levels (LH, FSH, and estradiol)
  (b) Males
    i) Spermatogenesis is an ongoing event; cellular damage occurs repeatedly because of continual cycling and dividing.
    ii) Azoospermia
    iii) Oligospermia (may last up to three years or never return to pretreatment levels)
4. Collaborative management
  a) Interventions prior to chemotherapy
    (1) Males should be encouraged to preserve sperm at a sperm bank before starting treatment. However, patients should be advised that men are likely to have a low sperm count before undergoing treatment.
    (2) Although expensive and not always successful, females should be informed that opportunities to bank oocytes or cryopreserve embryos are available in research settings (Kaempfer, Wiley, Hoffman, & Rhodes, 1985; Schilsky & Erlichman, 1982).
  b) Interventions during and after chemotherapy
    (1) Males
      (a) Monitor serum FSH and testosterone levels.
      (b) Obtain semen analysis to evaluate fertility.
      (c) Testosterone replacement has been tried with some

Table 24. Cancer-Associated Drugs That Affect Sexual and Reproductive Function

Agent	Complication
Antiemetics/sedatives/tranquilizers Prochlorperazine Chlorpromazine Diazepam Lorazepam Metoclopramide Scopolamine	Sedation, orgasm without ejaculation, impotence, decreased sexual interest, decreased intensity of orgasm
Antihistamines Diphenhydramine	Sedation, decreased sexual interest
Antidepressants Amitriptyline Imipramine	Impotence, altered libido
Narcotics Morphine Hydromorphone Codeine	Decreased libido, sedation, impaired potency
Miscellaneous Ketoconazole Cimetidine	Decreased libido Impotence
Corticosteroids	(See Table 23)

Note. From "Sexual and Reproductive Dysfunction," by L. Krebs, in S.L. Groenwald, M.H. Frogge, M. Goodman, and C.H. Yarbro (Eds.), Cancer Nursing: Principles and Practice (3rd ed.), p. 706, Boston: Jones & Bartlett. Copyright 1993 by Jones & Bartlett. Adapted with permission.

success (Kaempfer et al., 1985; Schilsky & Erlichman, 1982). Positive effects include maintenance of bone and muscle mass in older patients (Kaiser, 1992).

(2) Females

(a) Water-based lubricants or estrogen supplements may help to decrease vaginal dryness.

(b) Encourage discussion of concerns with partner and nurse or physician. Counseling or hormone supplements (e.g., testosterone) may be considered for decreased libido.

(c) Suggest using relaxation exercises or modifying positions in the event of painful intercourse. (If pain is caused by vaginal dryness, relaxation exercises will not help.)

5. Patient education and counseling

a) Adhere to general principles.

(1) Provide an unbiased, sexually neutral environment that promotes open discussion of the topic.

(2) Identify whether sexual issues pose a problem to the patient and his or her partner. The patient may focus on issues more over time.

(3) Listen for specific values and concerns the patient may have.

b) Explain the implications of treatment(s) on sexuality and that adequate sexual functioning may be central to a person's sexuality.

c) Provide information related to contraception.

d) Discourage pregnancy during the treatment period and discuss the timing of pregnancy after treatment.

e) Advise the patient of potential long-term side effects and the possibility of regaining reproductive function.

f) Encourage communication between the patient and significant other.

L. Cutaneous reactions (see Table 25)

1. Pathophysiology: Exact mechanism is unknown.

2. Incidence

a) Frequency varies according to reaction.

b) Common reactions include rash and alopecia.

3. Assessment, management, and education (see Table 25)

M. Ocular toxicity

1. Pathophysiology

a) Exact etiology is poorly understood in most cases.

b) The effects span a wide range of disorders, including inflammatory conditions (e.g., uveitis, conjunctivitis, keratitis, blepharitis, iritis), cataract formation, lid and lacrimation disorders, and neurologic injuries.

c) Problem significance (These ocular effects are rare and, in some cases, have only been seen in patients receiving very high-dose chemotherapy.)

(1) Ocular changes may go unnoticed until damage is irreversible.

(2) Ocular signs and symptoms may precede the development of peripheral neuropathies and, thus, may be an important marker of neurologic status.

(3) Ocular changes may be incorrectly attributed to the aging process.

(4) The incidence of ocular toxicities may be increased with administration of higher doses of antineoplastics, which has been made possible by the use of hematopoietic CSFs (Bull & Ruiz, 1992).

2. Incidence: Varies according to drug classification, dosage, and route of administration (see Table 26)

3. Assessment

a) Risk factors

(1) Causal relationships between agents and ocular toxicities are difficult to establish. Risk factors are equally difficult to establish.

(2) With cisplatin, the risk for ocular toxicity is greater in females and elderly patients.

b) Clinical manifestations (see Table 26)

c) Physical assessment

Table 25. Cutaneous Reactions

Cutaneous Reaction	Pathophysiology	Incidence	Nursing Assessment	Risk Factors	Collaborative Management
Acral erythema 1. A painful, erythematous, and edematous rash on the palmar surfaces of the hands and plantar surfaces of the feet 2. General progression to bulla formation, desquamation, and re-epithelialization (Kerker & Hood, 1989; Kroll, Koller, Kaled, & Dreizen, 1989; Shall, Lucus, Whittaker, & Holt., 1988)	1. Exact mechanism unknown 2. May represent accumulation of chemotherapeutic agents in eccrine glands (palms and soles contain vast eccrine glands) 3. May represent direct chemotoxicity on dermal vasculature	1. 80% in patients receiving high-dose cytarabine (Kroll et al., 1989) 2. Incidence increased when therapy includes continuous therapy of 5-fluorouracil and other drugs indicated in acral erythema	1. Assess potential for acral erythema from risk factors. 2. Inspect palmar and plantar surfaces frequently for sensation, color, movement. 3. Monitor for signs and symptoms of infection related to condition (Richards & Wujcik, 1992). 4. Assess for pain/discomfort.	1. High-dose cytarabine chemotherapy 2. Also associated with bleomycin, fluorouracil, doxorubicin, cyclophosphamide, methotrexate, and mercaptopurine	1. Apply cold compresses to affected areas to relieve pain. 2. Elevate the affected areas to reduce edema. 3. Apply steroid creams. 4. Administer pyridoxine 50 mg three times per day (Vukelja, Lombardo, James, & Weiss, 1989).
Hyperpigmentation 1. Increased amounts of epidermal melanin without dermal deposition in the skin, hair, nails, mucous membranes, and teeth (Kerker & Hood, 1989)	1. Exact mechanism unknown 2. May result from direct stimulation of the melanocyte 3. May impede melanin transfer within keratinocytes (DeSpain, 1992a; Kerker & Hood, 1989)	1. Exact incidence unknown; changes may be temporary or permanent. 2. Usually disappears within two to three months after completion of chemotherapy (Tenenbaum, 1989) 3. Causes no adverse effects	1. Skin assessment 2. Assess individual risk factors.	1. Increased incidence in dark-skinned individuals 2. May be associated with exogenous trauma/postinflammatory changes (i.e., dermatitis, photosensitive eruptions) 3. Increased in areas of vasodilation 4. Associated with many chemotherapeutic agents (highest incidence with alkylating agents and antitumor antibiotics)	1. Encourage patient to use sunscreens for photoprotection. 2. Avoid vasodilation during chemotherapy administration (avoid heating pads, warm compresses). 3. Treat inflammatory skin changes (e.g., dermatitis) promptly to avoid postinflammatory hyperpigmentation.
Inflammation of keratoses 1. Inflammation of actinic keratoses 2. Pruritus and erythema may be noted adjacent to previous actinic keratoses (DeSpain, 1992a; Kerker & Hood, 1989).	1. Exact etiology unknown 2. May be the result of DNA toxicity of the keratinocytic lesions	Incidence unknown	1. Skin assessment of potentially affected areas of actinic keratoses (face, arms, hands, and upper chest)	1. History of actinic keratoses 2. Highest incidence with fluorouracil chemotherapy (Schlang & Curtin, 1977) 3. Associated with various chemotherapeutic agents: dacarbazine, dactinomycin, doxorubicin, pentostatin (Camisa, Grever, & Bouroncle, 1985; Hardwick & Murray, 1986; Johnson, Rapini, & Duvic, 1987)	1. Report skin changes to the physician. 2. Distinguish inflammatory reaction from an allergic drug reaction. 3. Monitor for local and systemic signs of infection.
Nail changes 1. May include hyperpigmentation, discoloration, transverse banding, nail grooving (Beau's lines), and onycholysis (partial separation of nail plate from bed) (DeSpain, 1992a)	1. Hyperpigmentation due to melanin deposition in the nail plate	Incidence unknown	1. Assess nails prior to chemotherapy, and note any changes following administration.	1. May occur with bleomycin, cyclophosphamide, doxorubicin, floxuridine, fluorouracil, procarbazine, and taxotere	1. Instruct patient of potential nail changes, occurring 5–10 weeks after chemotherapy is initiated.

(Continued on next page)

Table 25. Cutaneous Reactions (Continued)

Cutaneous Reaction	Pathophysiology	Incidence	Nursing Assessment	Risk Factors	Collaborative Management
Nail changes (cont.)	2. Beau's lines due to chemotherapeutic toxicity of nail matrix	Incidence unknown	2. Assess individual risk factors.		2. Inform patient that changes are usually temporary (Tenenbaum, 1989). With taxotere, nails eventually fall off.
Neutrophilic eccrine hydradenitis (NEH) 1. Tender, erythematous macules, papules, and plaques on the trunk, neck, and extremities (Kerker & Hood, 1989) 2. Also may consist of hyperpigmented papules (Kerker & Hood, 1989) 3. May be associated with a fever without documented infection (DeSpain, 1992a)	1. Exact etiology unknown 2. May represent a direct toxicity of the eccrine coils (Flynn, Harrist, Murphy, Loss, & Moschella, 1984; Harrist, Fine, Berman, Murphy, & Mihm, 1982)	Incidence unknown	1. Perform skin assessment with specific attention to the trunk, neck, and extremities. 2. Assess for elevated temperature.	1. Possibly associated with acute leukemia 2. Most commonly occurs with cytosine arabinoside and bleomycin	1. Assess for other potential sources of infection when fever is present. 2. Inform the patient that the lesions and associated fever will resolve spontaneously.
Radiation enhancement 1. A synergistic effect of concurrent radiation therapy and chemotherapy, which augments the effects of the radiation 2. May involve cutaneous edema, erythema, blisters, erosions, ulceration, or hyperpigmentation in radiated field (DeSpain, 1992a)	1. Exact etiology unknown 2. Related to specific chemotherapeutic agents that intercalate with DNA and prevent cellular repair of radiation injury	Incidence unknown	1. Perform skin assessment before radiation is initiated and daily thereafter. 2. Assess for individual risk factors. 3. Assess affected area for signs of local infection.	1. May only occur if chemotherapy is administered within one week of radiation therapy 2. Associated chemotherapy: dactinomycin, doxorubicin, bleomycin, hydroxyurea, fluorouracil, and methotrexate (Jaffe, Paed, & Farber, 1973; Phillips & Fu, 1977)	1. Instruct patient to avoid trauma and irritation to the affected area. 2. Apply cool, wet compresses with acute reaction. 3. Apply topical steroids as ordered. 4. Debride ulcerated areas and apply an antimicrobial ointment and a non-adherent dressing over area.
Radiation recall 1. An inflammatory reaction occurring in previously irradiated tissue 2. May occur in the skin, lung, gastrointestinal tract, and heart (DeSpain, 1992a)	Exact etiology unknown	Incidence unknown	See radiation enhancement, above	1. Most frequently associated with doxorubicin and dactinomycin.	See radiation enhancement, above
Hand-foot syndrome (acral erythema, palmarplantar erythrodysesthesia syndrome)	Exact etiology unknown; may be a vascular reaction	Depends on agent		1. Associated with continuous infusion of 5-fluorouracil, capecitabine (Xeloda®, Hoffmann–La Roche Inc., Nutley, NJ)	1. Pain control 2. Bag Balm® (Dairy Association Co., Inc., Lyndonville, VT)

Table 26. Ocular Toxicities of Chemotherapy

Chemotherapeutic Agent	Ocular Toxicity
Alkylating agents	
Nitrogen mustard	Intracarotid: ipsilateral necrotizing uveitis and necrotizing vasculitis of choroid (Anderson & Anderson, 1960)
Cyclophosphamide	Blurred vision (reversible), keratoconjunctivitis sicca, pinpoint pupils (parasympathomimetic effect of alkylating agents) (Jack & Hicks, 1981; Kende, Sirkin, Thomas, & Freeman, 1979)
Ifosfamide	Blurred vision (reversible), conjunctivitis (Choonara, Overend, & Bailey, 1987)
Cisplatin	IV: blurred vision, color blindness (blue-yellow), papilledema, neuro-retinal changes, optic neuritis, retrobulbar neuritis
	Intracarotid: ipsilateral visual loss (15%–60%) from retinal and/or optic nerve ischemia (preventable if catheter advanced beyond ophthalmic artery, but increases cerebral toxicity) (Becher, Schutt, Osieka, & Schmidt, 1980; Kupersmith et al., 1988; Ostrow, Hahn, Wiernik, & Richards, 1978; Wilding et al., 1985)
Chlorambucil	Keratitis, oculomotor disturbances, hemorrhagic retinopathy, papilledema (Vizel & Oster, 1982)
Busulfan	Cataract formation (Dahlgren, Holm, Svanborg, & Watz, 1972), nonspecific blurred vision and keratoconjunctivitis sicca (Fraunfelder & Meyer, 1987)
BCNU, CCNU, Methyl-CCNU	Penetrate the blood-brain retinal barriers (Bull & Ruiz, 1992)
Antimetabolites	
5-Fluorouracil	Blurred vision, periorbital edema, ocular pain, photophobia, excessive lacrimation, conjunctivitis, blepharitis, keratitis, punctalcanicular stenosis, oculomotor disturbances, ectropion, optic neuropathy (Caravella, Burns, & Zangmeister, 1981; Imperia, Lazarus, & Lass, 1989)
Cytosine arabinoside	IV: keratoconjunctivitis (keratitis incidence may be 100% with high dose) (Lass, Lazarus, Reed, & Herzig, 1982), ocular pain, photophobia, blurred vision Intrathecal: optic neuropathy (may be potentiated by cranial radiation therapy) (Hopen, Mondino, Johnson, & Chervenick, 1981; Margileth, Poplak, Pizzo, & Leventhal, 1977)
Fludarabine	Decreased visual acuity (most common presenting sign prior to development of progressive encephalopathy), diplopia, photophobia, papilledema, optic neuritis (Chun, Leyland-Jones, Caryk, & Hoth, 1986)
Methotrexate	IV: periorbital edema, photophobia, ocular pain/burning, blepharitis, conjunctivitis, reduced lacrimation Intrathecal/intracarotid: optic neuropathy (potentiated by cranial RT) (Doroshow et al., 1981)
Bromodeoxyuridine (BUdR)	Intracarotid with local radiation therapy: blepharitis, conjunctivitis, keratitis (Vander et al., 1990)
Antibiotics	
Doxorubicin	Increased lacrimation, conjunctivitis (Blum, 1975)
Mitomycin C	Blurred vision without ophthalmologic findings (not well established) (Vizel & Oster, 1982)
Mithramycin	Unique periorbital pallor (not well established) (Vizel & Oster, 1982)
Vinca alkaloids	Cranial nerve palsies (incidence as high as 50%) (Kaplan & Wiernik, 1982), ptosis, optic neuropathy/atrophy, decreased pupillary response to light, decreased visual acuity, poor color discrimination (Sandler, Tobin, & Henderson, 1969)
Miscellaneous	
Tamoxifen	Retinopathy, decreased visual acuity (Kaiser-Kupfer & Lippman, 1978)
Procarbazine	Retinal hemorrhage, photophobia, papilledema (Vizel & Oster, 1982)
Corticosteroids	Posterior subcapsular cataracts, glaucoma, retinal hemorrhage (Spaeth & Von Sallman, 1966), opportunistic eye infections
Biologic response modifiers	Optic disc edema with high doses, retinal vasculitis (Bull & Ruiz, 1982)

(1) Eyelid: Examine and palpate for signs of erythema and edema. Observe for exudate, crusting, and presence of ptosis. Observe condition of lashes.

(2) Conjunctiva: Invert lids and observe for hyperemia, edema, and discharge.

(3) Cornea: Observe for smooth appearance and clarity. Test corneal reflex by gently touching a cotton swab to the corneal surface.

(4) Iris: Observe the color. Pupil and iris margins should be clearly defined. Note pain and photophobia.

(5) Lacrimation: Note dryness, foreign body sensation, or excessive tearing. Use the Schirmer test (normal test: Wets Schirmer strip 1 mm/minute).

(6) Visual disturbances: Assess acuity using near vision card held at arm's length with glasses on. Obtain a chronology of visual changes, unilateral or bilateral involvement, and precipitating/relieving factors.

(7) Cranial nerves: Observe ocular alignment, light reflex, and extraocular muscles by having the patient follow finger movements in six planes.

4. Collaborative management

a) Refer the patient to an ophthalmologist if signs of toxicity are noted. Routine monitoring may be indicated for tamoxifen (Nolvadex®, Zeneca Pharmaceuticals, Wilmington, DE), particularly if the patient is participating in a clinical trial (e.g., some patients have reported seeing floaters).

b) Recommend eye drops and lubricants (e.g., dexamethasone eye drops 0.1% one drop twice a day) for cytarabine conjunctivitis.

c) Encourage the patient to undergo yearly eye examinations.

5. Patient education

a) Teach the patient self-examination and emphasize the importance of close monitoring and prompt reporting of any structural changes in eyelids, eyelashes, or vision.

b) Emphasize careful hygiene and hand-washing techniques to minimize cross-contamination. A demonstration of proper use of eye drops and lubricants may be useful.

N. Secondary malignancies

1. Pathophysiology (see Table 27)

a) Chemotherapy agents have long been recognized as having carcinogenic properties. Many act by producing DNA damage. Cytogenic and animal studies provide evidence that alkylating agents and anthracyclines have carcinogenic potential (Forbes, 1992). Topoisomerase-II inhibitors (e.g., topotecan, irinotecan) induce mutations in genes critical for cell survival (Smith, Rubinstein, & Ungerleider, 1994).

b) Secondary malignancies occur months to years after treatment for primary cancer and are occurring because of increased survival due to therapy improvements.

c) Both leukemias and solid tumors have been reported (Fraser & Tucker, 1988).

(1) Secondary leukemia related to alkylating agents is associated with preleukemic phase (Auclerc, Jacquillat, & Auclerc, 1979), chromosome 5 and 7 abnormalities (LeBeau et al., 1986), and poor prognosis (Kantaujian et al., l986; Pederson-Bjergaard, Philip, Larsen, Jensen, & Byrsting, 1990).

(2) Secondary leukemia related to epipodophyllotoxin (e.g., etoposide therapy) is associated with a short latency period, monocytic or myelomonocytic subtype, chromosome 9 and 11 abnormalities, and a good response to chemotherapy (Kumar, 1993; Smith et al., 1994).

d) Causes

(1) Single-agent chemotherapy

(a) Alkylating agents (e.g., melphalan, cyclophosphamide)

(b) Epipodophyllotoxins (e.g., etoposide [VePesid®,

Bristol-Myers Squibb On-
cology, Princeton, NJ],
teniposide [Vumon®,
Bristol-Myers Squibb On-
cology)
(2) Combination chemotherapy:
Use of multiple drugs (e.g.,
MOPP)
(3) Chemotherapy combined with
radiation therapy

(a) Chemotherapy and mantle
radiation therapy for
Hodgkin's lymphoma in-
creases the risk of breast
cancer for women (Boivin
et al., 1995; Hancock,
Tucker, & Hoppe, 1993).
(b) Chemotherapy and radiation therapy for testicular
cancer increase the risk of

Table 27. Secondary Malignancies Related to Chemotherapy

Secondary Malignancy	Primary Malignancy Factors	Occurrence	Risk Factors
Leukemia	Breast	No significant time to occurrence	Melphalan-based adjuvant therapy
	Gastrointestinal (colon, gastric, rectal)	Unknown	Methyl-lomustine (CCNU) (Boice et al., 1983)
	Hodgkin's disease (stage not a factor)	Within 10 years after treatment	Mechlorethamine, Oncovin® (vincristine), procarbazine, prednisone (MOPP) (Boivin et al., 1995; Tucker, Coleman, Cox, Varghese, & Rosenberg, 1988)
	Small cell lung	No specific time to occurrence	Busulfan, cyclophosphamide, CCNU, procarbazine, etoposide (Kumar, 1993)
	Non-small cell lung	No specific time to occurrence	Cisplatin, etoposide (Chak, Sikic, Tucker, Horns, & Cox, 1984; Stott, Fox, Girling, Stephens, & Galton, 1977)
	Multiple myeloma	No specific time to occurrence	Melphalan (Bergsagel et al., 1979)
	Non-Hodgkin's lymphoma	No specific time to occurrence	Carmustine (BCNU), mechlorethamine, cyclophosphamide, vincristine (Gomez, Aggarwal, & Han, 1982); combined chemotherapy and radiation
	Ovarian	Five to seven years after treatment	Cyclophosphamide, melphalan > 700 mg (Greene et al., 1986)
	Polycythemia vera[a]	No specific time to occurrence	Chlorambucil
	Testicular	Within three years	Etoposide > 2 g/m^2 weekly or twice weekly and combination chemotherapy (Bokemeyer & Schmoll, 1995; Kumar, 1993)
Non-Hodgkin's lymphoma	Hodgkin's disease	No specific time to occurrence	Alkylating agents (Beaty et al., 1995; Fraser & Tucker, 1988)
Endometrial	Breast	Within eight years after starting treatment	Tamoxifen (Fisher et al., 1994; Rutqvist et al., 1995)
Bladder	Various cancers[b]	No specific time to occurrence	Cyclophosphamide (Travis et al., 1995; Wall & Clausen, 1975)
Breast	Hodgkin's disease	10–20 years in females under age 30 treated with mantle-field irradiation	Mantle radiation therapy and chemotherapy (Boivin et al., 1995; Hancock, Tucker, & Hoppe, 1993)
Respiratory and intrathoracic (including lung)	Hodgkin's disease	Five years; increases with time	Thoracic radiation therapy and chemotherapy (Boivin et al., 1995; Van Leeuwen et al., 1994)
Gastrointestinal	Testicular	Elevated risk factor of 2–3 within 10–20 years	Radiation therapy (Bokemeyer & Schmoll, 1995)

[a] Has potential to transform to leukemia as disease-related phenomenon (Berk et al., 1981)
[b] Strong dose-response relationship reported

solid tumors within the radiation field (Bokemeyer & Schmoll, 1995).

(4) Hormonal therapy: Tamoxifen is associated with the secondary development of endometrial cancer (Fisher et al., 1994).

2. Incidence
   a) Frequently reported as absolute risk over the comparison population (i.e., three more cancers per 100 patients).
   b) Leukemia risk peaks within 10 years of primary therapy (Beaty et al., 1995; Forbes, 1992; Smith et al., 1994).
   c) Solid tumor risk continues more than 10 years after primary therapy (Beaty et al., 1995; Forbes, 1992; Travis et al., 1995).
   d) Secondary malignancies have been reported in patients receiving chemotherapy for diseases other than cancer.

3. Assessment
   a) Risk factors
      (1) Genetic predisposition: New research in cloning and sequencing genes may provide additional information about relationships between genetic predisposition, cancer treatment, and secondary malignancies (Malkin et al., 1992).
      (2) Gender: Females treated for Hodgkin's disease are at a greater risk for secondary cancers, even when those with breast cancer were removed from analysis (Beaty et al., 1995; Boivin et al., 1995)
      (3) Age at cancer diagnosis: Adolescents (at least age 10 at diagnosis) treated for Hodgkin's disease are at a greater risk for secondary cancers than preadolescents (Beaty et al., 1995)
      (4) Multiple drug regimens (four or more) increase risk over combinations of three or less drugs (Glicksman et al., 1982).
      (5) Schedule of therapy administration: Epipodophyllotoxins (e.g., etoposide, teniposide) administered on a weekly or

twice-weekly schedule are associated with a greater risk of leukemia than when administered daily for four days (Smith et al., 1994).

4. Collaborative management
   a) Leukemia
      (1) Assessment should include looking for signs and symptoms of anemia, bleeding, or frequent infections.
      (2) Review CBC, looking for anemia, abnormal WBC count, or thrombocytopenia. If abnormal, consider bone marrow aspiration and biopsy with cytogenetics.
   b) Breast: mammography screening and diligent breast exam beginning 10 years after mantle radiation therapy
   c) Endometrial
      (1) Annual gynecological examinations should be performed.
      (2) Any abnormal vaginal bleeding should be investigated by endometrial biopsy (American College of Obstetricians and Gynecologists, 1996).

5. Patient education
   a) Patient education should include information about the risks of secondary malignancies, time to onset, signs and symptoms of secondary cancers, and the importance of follow-up visits.
   b) Professional education should include the above, with special efforts to educate primary-care professionals who may follow patients beyond the years that oncologists typically follow patients.

The Clinical Practicum

I. Course Description

The clinical practicum allows the nurse to apply the knowledge gained in the didactic component to direct patient-care situations. Emphasis is placed on the clinical skills that a nurse must demonstrate prior to being considered competent to administer chemotherapy.

II. Course Objectives

At the completion of the clinical practicum, the nurse will be able to demonstrate the following behaviors (see Appendix 5).

A. Demonstrate safety and proficiency in the preparation, storage, transport, handling, administration, and disposal of chemotherapy drugs and equipment.
B. Identify appropriate physical and laboratory assessments for specific chemotherapy agents.
C. Demonstrate skill in venipuncture, including vein selection and sterile technique.
D. Demonstrate skill in the care and use of various VADs.
E. Identify patient and family educational needs in relation to specific chemotherapy agents.
F. Identify acute local or systemic reactions as a result of extravasation or anaphylaxis in association with specific chemotherapy drugs and appropriate interventions.
G. Demonstrate proficiency in the safe administration of chemotherapy and disposal of chemotherapy wastes and equipment.
H. Verbalize knowledge of institutional policies and procedures regarding chemotherapy administration.
I. Document pertinent information in the medical record.

III. Clinical Activities

A. The nurse should be supervised by a qualified preceptor to ensure safe practice.
B. The preceptor and the nurse should establish specific objectives at the beginning of the clinical practicum. Ideally, the nurse and the preceptor should select a specific population of patients, and the nurse should assume responsibility for planning the care for these patients with supervision by the preceptor.
C. The length of time spent in the supervised clinical practicum should be individualized, depending on the nurse's ability and skill in meeting the specific objectives and institutional standards.
D. Once the nurse becomes proficient and independent in administering nonvesicants, progression to vesicant administration can occur.
E. The nurse should verbalize to the preceptor potential adverse reactions, side effects, toxicities, and measures to prevent and/or manage these reactions.

F. Various clinical settings can be used for the nurse to demonstrate knowledge of chemotherapy administration. It may not be realistic for all settings or agencies to provide chemotherapy education and training. Other recommendations include the following.
   1. Contracting with major institutions to credential nurses for specific needs (e.g., vesicant, nonvesicant, IV push, short infusion, continuous infusion)
   2. Creating a simulated lab to substitute for the clinical component when patients are not available

IV. Evaluation

An evaluation tool based on the practicum course objectives should be used to determine the following.

A. The nurse's knowledge of chemotherapy drugs and the associated nursing implications
B. The nurse's knowledge of the necessary technical skills required for the administration of chemotherapy agents (e.g., venipuncture, VAD access and management, indwelling catheter management)
C. The nurse's knowledge of patient education, which should be initiated based on the chemotherapy administered
D. The nurse's knowledge of steps to be taken in the event of an untoward response following chemotherapy administration (e.g., anaphylaxis, hypersensitivity reaction, extravasation)
E. Following successful completion of the clinical practicum, the nurse should complete a skills inventory to demonstrate his or her ability to perform the four criteria described above (see Appendices 5 and 6). This can be done in a simulated setting (e.g., skills lab) or as a precepted experience in the clinical setting. It is recommended that the learner administer at least three chemotherapy agents under the supervision of trained personnel. Two should be administered by an IV push—the first should be a nonvesicant agent, and the second should be a vesicant agent. Annual evaluation is recommended, and the content should, at a minimum, emphasize any new information available.

References

Abeloff, M. (1995). Vinorelbine (Navelbine) in the treatment of breast cancer: A summary. *Seminars in Oncology, 22*(6 Suppl. 5), 1–4.

Aistars, J. (1987). Fatigue in the cancer patient: A conceptual approach to a clinical problem. *Oncology Nursing Forum, 14*(6), 25–30.

Ajani, J.A., Dodd, L.G., Daugherty, K., Warkentin, D., & Ilson, D.H. (1994). Taxol-induced soft-tissue injury secondary to extravasation: Characterization by histopathology and clinical course. *Journal of the National Cancer Institute, 86,* 51–53.

Akhtar, S.S., Salim, K.P., & Bano, Z.A. (1993). Symptomatic cardiotoxicity with high-dose 5-fluorouracil infusion: A prospective study. *Oncology, 50,* 441–444.

Alberts, D.S., & Dorr, R.T. (1991). Case report: Topical DMSO for mitomycin-C-induced skin ulceration. *Oncology Nursing Forum, 18,* 693–695.

Allen, A. (1992). The cardiotoxicity of chemotherapeutic drugs. In M.C. Perry (Ed.), *The chemotherapy source book* (pp. 582–597). Baltimore: Williams & Wilkins.

Aly, R., Bayles, C., & Malbach, H. (1988). Restriction of bacterial growth under commercial catheter dressings. *American Journal of Infection Control, 16*(3), 95–100.

American College of Obstetricians and Gynecologists. (1996, February). Tamoxifen and endometrial cancer. *Committee Opinions,* No. 169, pp. 1–3.

American Nurses Association and Oncology Nursing Society. (1996). *Statement on the scope and standards of oncology nursing practice.* Washington, DC: American Nurses Publishing.

American Pain Society. (1992). *Principles of analgesic use in the treatment of acute pain and cancer pain.* Skokie: IL: Author.

American Society of Hospital Pharmacists. (1990). *ASHP technical assistance bulletin on handling cytotoxic and hazardous drugs.* Bethesda, MD: Author.

Anand, A.J. (1994). Fluorouracil cardiotoxicity. *Annals of Pharmacotherapy, 28,* 374–378.

Anderson, B., & Anderson, B., Jr. (1960). Necrotizing uveitis incident to perfusion of intracranial malignancies with nitrogen mustard or related compounds. *Transactions of the American Ophthalmological Society, 58,* 95–104.

Anderson, N., & Lokich, J.J. (1994). Cancer chemotherapy and infusional scheduling. *Oncology, 8*(5), 99–111.

Anderson, R., Dorr, R.T., Finley, R., Green, L., Koeller, J., & Phillips, N. (1993). *Practical guidelines for dispensing oral anticancer drugs.* Princeton, NJ: Bristol-Myers Squibb.

Andrykowski, M.A. (1988). Defining anticipatory nausea and vomiting: Differences among cancer chemotherapy patients who report pretreatment nausea. *Journal of Behavioral Medicine, 11*(1), 59–69.

Arbuck, S.G., Adams, J., & Strauss, H. (1992). A reassessment of cardiac toxicity associated with Taxol. Abstract presented at Second National Cancer Institute Workshop on Taxol and Taxus, Sept. 23–24, Alexandria, VA.

Arlin, Z.A., Sklaroff, R.B., Gee, T.S., Kempin, S.J., Howard, J., Clarkson, B.D., & Young, C.W. (1980). Phase I and II trial of 4'(9-acridinylamino) methanesulfon-m-anisidide in patients with acute leukemia. *Cancer Research, 40,* 3304–3306.

Auclerc, G., Jacquillat, C., & Auclerc, M.F. (1979). Post-therapeutic acute leukemia. *Cancer, 44,* 2017–2025.

Avis, K.E., & Levchuk, J.W. (1984). Special considerations in the use of vertical laminar-flow workbenches. *American Journal of Hospital Pharmacy, 41*(1), 81–87.

Bach, F., Videbaek, C., Holst-Christensen, J., & Boesby, S. (1991). Cytostatic extravasation: A serious complication of long-term venous access. *Cancer, 68,* 538–539.

Baker, B.W., Wilson, C.L., Davis, A.L., Spearing, R.L., Hart, D.N., Heaton, D.C., & Beard, M.E. (1991). Busulfan/cyclophosphamide conditioning for bone marrow transplantation may lead to failure of hair regrowth. *Bone Marrow Transplantation, 7*(1), 43–47.

Barnett, M.J., Richards, M.A., Ganesan, T.S. Waxman, J.H., Smith, B.F., Butler, M.G., Rohatiner, A.Z., Slevin, M.L., & Lister, T.A. (1985). Central nervous system toxicity of high-dose cytosine arabinoside. *Seminars in Oncology Nursing, 12*(2 Suppl. 3), 227–232.

Barr, R., Furlong, W., Henwood, J., Feeny, D., Wegener, J., Walker, I., & Brain, M. (1996). Economic evaluation of allogeneic bone marrow transplantation: A rudimentary model to generate estimates for the timely formulation of clinical policy. *Journal of Clinical Oncology, 14,* 1413–1420.

Barton-Burke, M., Wilkes, G.M., & Ingwersen, K. (1992). *Chemotherapy care plans: Designs for nursing care.* Boston: Jones & Bartlett.

Barton-Burke, M., Wilkes, G.M., Ingwersen, K.C., Bean, C.K., & Berg, D. (1996). *Cancer chemotherapy: A nursing process approach* (2nd ed.). Boston: Jones & Bartlett.

Basch, A. (1987). Changes in elimination associated with cancer. *Seminars in Oncology Nursing, 3,* 287–292.

Baxley, K.O., Erdman, L.K., Henry, E.B., & Roof, B.J. (1984). Alopecia: Effect on cancer patients' body image. *Cancer Nursing, 7,* 499–503.

Beaty, O., Hudson, M.M., Greenwald, C., Luo, X., Fang, L., Wilimas, J.A., Thompson, E.I., Kun, L.E., & Pratt, C.B. (1995). Subsequent malignancies in children and adolescents after treatment for Hodgkin's disease. *Journal of Clinical Oncology, 13,* 603–609.

Beauchamp, T.L., & Childress, J.F. (1994). *Principles of biomedical ethics* (4th ed.). New York: Oxford University Press.

Becher, R., Schutt, P., Osieka, R., & Schmidt, C.G. (1980). Peripheral neuropathy and ophthalmologic toxicity after treatment with cis-dichlorodiaminoplatinum II. *Journal of Cancer Research and Clinical Oncology, 96*(2), 219–221.

Beck, S.A., & Tisdale, M.J. (1987). Production of lipolytic and proteolytic factors by a murine tumor producing cachexia in the host. *Cancer Research, 47,* 5919–5923.

Beck, S.L. (1992). Prevention and management of oral complications in the cancer patient. *Current Issues in Cancer Nursing Practice Updates, 1*(6), 1–12.

Bellone, J.D. (1981). Treatment of vincristine extravasation [Letter to the editor]. *JAMA, 245,* 343.

Bender, C. (1998). Implications of antineoplastic therapy for nursing. In J.K. Itano & K.N. Taoka (Eds.), *Core curriculum for oncology nursing* (3rd ed.) (pp. 641–656). Philadelphia: Saunders.

Benoliel, J.Q. (1993). The moral context of oncology nursing. *Oncology Nursing Forum, 20*(Suppl. 10), 5–12.

Bergsagel, D.E., Bailey, A.J., Langley, G.R., MacDonald, R.N., White, D.F., & Miller, A.B. (1979). The chemotherapy of plasma-cell myeloma and the incidence of acute leukemia. *New England Journal of Medicine, 301,* 743–748.

Berk, P.D., Goldberg, J.D., Silverstein, M.N., Weinfeld, A., Donovan, P.B., Ellis, J.T., Landaw, S.A., Laszlo, J., Najean, Y., Pisciotta, A.V., & Wasserman, L.R. (1981). Increased incidence of acute leukemia in polycythemia vera associated with chlorambucil therapy. *New England Journal of Medicine, 304,* 441–447.

Berry, D.L, Dodd, M.J., Hinds, P.S., & Ferrell, B.R. (1996). Informed consent: Process and clinical issues. *Oncology Nursing Forum, 23,* 507–512.

Bertelli, G. (1994). Prevention and management of extravasation of cytotoxic drugs. *Drug Safety, 12,* 245–255.

Bertino, J.R., & O'Keefe, P. (1992). Barriers and strategies for effective chemotherapy. *Seminars in Oncology Nursing, 8,* 77–82.

Beutler, E. (1993). Platelet transfusions: The 20,000/uL trigger. *Blood, 81,* 1411–1413.

Blackburn, G.L., Maini, B.S., Bistrian, B.S., Wade, J.E., & Tayek, J.A. (1987). Surgical nutrition. In S.L. Halpern (Ed.), *Quick reference to clinical nutrition* (2nd ed.) (pp. 170–194). Phildelphia: Lippincott.

Blecke, C. (1989). Home chemotherapy safety procedures. *Oncology Nursing Forum, 16,* 719–721.

Blesch, K., Paice, J., Wickham, R., Harte, N., Schnoor, D., Purl, S., Rehwalt, M., Kopp, P., Manson, S., Coveny, S., McHale, M., & Cahill, M. (1991). Correlates of fatigue in people with breast or lung cancer. *Oncology Nursing Forum, 18,* 81–87.

Blesch, K.S. (1988). The normal physiological changes of aging and their impact on the response to cancer treatment. *Seminars in Oncology Nursing, 4,* 178–188.

Blum, R. (1975). An overview of studies with Adriamycin in the United States. *Cancer Chemotherapy Reports, 6,* 247–251.

Blum, R.H., Carter, S.K., & Agre, K. (1973). A clinical review of bleomycin—A new antineoplastic agent. *Cancer, 31,* 903–914.

Boice, J.D., Jr., Greene, M.H., Killen, J.Y., Jr., Ellenberg, S.S., Keehn, R.J., McFadden, E., Chen, T.T., & Fraumeni, J.F., Jr. (1983). Leukemia and preleukemia after adjuvant treatment of gastrointestinal cancer with semustine (methyl-CCNU). *New England Journal of Medicine, 309,* 1079–1084.

Boivin, J., Hutchinson, G.B., Zauber, A., Bernstein, L., Davis, F., Michel, R., Zanke, B., Tan, C., Fuller, L., Mauch, D., & Ultman, J. (1995). Incidence of second cancers in patients treated for Hodgkin's disease. *Journal of the National Cancer Institute, 87,* 732–741.

Bokemeyer, C., & Schmoll, H.J. (1995). Treatment of testicular cancer and the development of secondary malignancies. *Journal of Clinical Oncology, 13,* 283–292.

Bonadonna, G., Valagussa, P., Rossi, A., Brambilla, C., Zambetti, M., & Veronesi, U. (1985). Ten-year experience with CMF-based adjuvant chemotherapy in resectable breast cancer. *Breast Cancer Research Treatment, 5,* 95–115.

Bonadonna, G., Zambetti, M., & Valagussa, P. (1995). Sequential or alternating doxorubicin and CMF regimens in breast cancer with more than three positive nodes: Ten-year results. *JAMA, 273,* 542–547.

Bookman, M.A., Kloth, D.D, Kover, P.E., Smolinski, S., & Ozols, R.F. (1997). Short-course intravenous prophylaxis for paclitaxel-related hypersensitivity reactions. *Annals of Oncology, 8,* 611–614.

Boyle, D.M., & Engelking, C. (1995). Vesicant extravasation: Myths and realities. *Oncology Nursing Forum, 22,* 57–67.

Broder, L.E., & Carter, S.K. (1973). Pancreatic islet cell carcinoma, II: Results of therapy with streptozotocin in 52 patients. *Annals of Internal Medicine, 79*(1), 108–118.

Brophy, L., & Sharp, E. (1991). Physical symptoms of combination biotherapy: A quality-of-life issue. *Oncology Nursing Forum, 18*(Suppl. 1), 25–30.

Brothers, T.E., Von Moll, L.K., Niederhuber, J.E., Roberts, J.A., Walker-Andrews, S., & Ensminger, W.D. (1988). Experience with subcutaneous ports in three hundred patients. *Surgery, Gynecology & Obstetrics, 166,* 295–301.

Brown, J., & Hogan, C. (1990). Chemotherapy. In S.L. Groenwald, M.H. Frogge, M. Goodman, & C.H. Yarbro (Eds.), *Cancer nursing: Principles and practice* (pp. 230–284). Boston: Jones & Bartlett.

Bull, J.M., & Ruiz, R.S. (1992). Ocular complications of systemic cancer therapy. *The Cancer Bulletin, 44,* 395–403.

Burchenal, J.H. (1977). The historical development of cancer chemotherapy. *Seminars in Oncology, 4,* 135–148.

Burns, L. (1992). The cardiotoxicity of chemotherapeutic drugs. In M.C. Perry (Ed.), *The chemotherapy source book* (pp. 582–597). Baltimore: Williams & Wilkins.

Calvert, A.H., Newell, D.R., & Gore, M.E. (1992). Future directions with carboplatin: Can therapeutic monitoring, high-dose administration, and hematologic support with growth factors expand the spectrum compared with cisplatin? *Seminars in Oncology, 19*(Suppl. 2), 155–163.

Camisa, C., Grever, M.R., & Bouroncle, B. (1985). Deoxycoformycin: A new chemotherapeutic agent of interest to dermatologists [Letter to the editor]. *Journal of the Academy of Dermatology, 12,* 1108–1109.

Camp-Sorrell, D. (Ed.). (1996). *Access device guidelines: Recommendations for nursing practice and education.* Pittsburgh: Oncology Nursing Press, Inc., a subsidiary of the Oncology Nursing Society.

Camp-Sorrell, D. (1997). Chemotherapy: Toxicity management. In S.L. Groenwald, M.H. Frogge, M. Goodman, & C.H. Yarbo (Eds.), *Cancer nursing: Principles and practice* (4th ed.) (pp. 385–425). Boston: Jones & Bartlett.

Capizzi, R.L., Bertino, J.R., & Handschumacher, R.E. (1970). L-asparaginase. *Annual Review of Medicine, 21,* 433–444.

Caravella, L.P., Jr., Burns, J.A., & Zangmeister, M. (1981). Punctal-canalicular stenosis related to systemic fluorouracil therapy. *Archives of Ophthalmology, 99,* 284–286.

Carlson, R.W. (1992). Reducing the cardiotoxicity of the anthracyclines. *Oncology, 6*(6), 95–108.

Cavalli, F., Tschopp, L., Sonntag, R.W., & Zimmerman, A. (1978). A case of liver toxicity following cis-dichlorodiammineplatinum (ii) treatment. *Cancer Treatment Reports, 62,* 2125–2126.

Ceci, G., Bella, M., Melissari, M., Gabrielli, M., Bocchi, P., & Cocconi, G. (1988). Fatal hepatic vascular toxicity of DTIC: Is it really a rare event? *Cancer, 61,* 1988–1991.

Chak, L.Y., Sikic, B.I., Tucker, M.A., Horns, R.C., Jr., & Cox, R.S. (1984). Increased incidence of acute nonlymphocytic leukemia following therapy in patients with small cell carcinoma of the lung. *Journal of Clinical Oncology, 2,* 385–390.

Choonara, I.A., Overend, M., & Bailey, C.C. (1987). Blurring of vision due to ifosfamide [Letter to the editor]. *Cancer Chemotherapy and Pharmacology, 20,* 349.

Chrystal, C. (1997). Administering continuous vesicant chemotherapy in the ambulatory setting. *Journal of Intravenous Nursing, 20*(2), 78–88.

Chun, H.G., Leyland-Jones, B.R., Caryk, S.M., & Hoth, D.F. (1986). Central nervous system toxicity of fludarabine phosphate. *Cancer Treatment Reports, 70,* 1225–1228.

Ciesielski-Carlucci, C., Leong, P., & Jacobs, C. (1997). Case report of anaphylaxis from cisplatin/paclitaxel and a review of their hypersensitivity reaction profiles. *American Journal of Clinical Oncology, 20,* 373–375.

Cleri, L.B. (1995). Serotonin antagonists: State of the art management of chemotherapy-induced emesis. *Oncology Nursing: Treatment and Support, 2*(1), 1–19.

Cloak, M.M., Connor, T.H., Stevens, K.R., Theiss, J., Alt, J., Matney, T., & Anderson, R. (1985). Occupational exposure of nursing personnel to antineoplastic agents. *Oncology Nursing Forum, 12*(5), 33–39.

Conn, C. (1993). The importance of syringe size when using implanted vascular access devices. *NAVAN, 3*(1), 11–18.

Conrad, K.J. (1986). Cerebellar toxicities associated with cytosine arabinoside: A nursing perspective. *Oncology Nursing Forum, 13*(5), 57–59.

Conrad, K.J., & Horrell, C.J. (Eds.). (1995). *Biotherapy: Recommendations for nursing course content and clinical practicum.* Pittsburgh: Oncology Nursing Society.

Cotanch, P.H. (1991). Use of nonpharmacological techniques to prevent chemotherapy-related nausea and vomiting. *Recent Results in Cancer Research, 121,* 101–107.

Crawford, J., Ozer, H., Stroller, R., Johnson, D., Lyman, G., Tabbara, I., Kris, M., Grous, J., Picozzi, V., Rausch, G., Smith, R., Gradishar, W., Yahanda, A., Vincent, M., Stewart, M., & Glaspy, J. (1991). Reduction by granulocyte colony-stimulating factor of fever and neutropenia induced by chemotherapy in patients with small cell lung cancer. *New England Journal of Medicine, 325,* 164–170.

Creaven, P.J., & Mihich, E. (1977). The clinical toxicity of anticancer drugs and its prediction. *Seminars in Oncology, 4,* 147–163.

Cubeddu, L.X. (1992). Mechanisms by which cancer chemotherapeutic drugs induce emesis [Review]. *Seminars in Oncology, 19*(Suppl. 15), 2–13.

Curran, C.F., Luce, J.K., & Page, J.A. (1990). Doxorubicin-associated flare reactions. *Oncology Nursing Forum, 17,* 387–389.

Dahlgren, S., Holm, G., Svanborg, N., & Watz, R. (1972). Clinical and morphological side-effects of busulfan (Myleran) treatment. *Acta Medica Scandinavica, 192*(1–2), 129–135.

Derogatis, L.R., & Kourlesis, S.M. (1981). An approach to evaluation of sexual problems in the cancer patient. *CA: A Cancer Journal for Clinicians, 31,* 46–50.

DeSpain, J.D. (1992a). Dermatologic toxicity. In M.C. Perry (Ed.), *The chemotherapy source book* (pp. 531–547). Baltimore: Williams & Wilkins.

DeSpain, J.D. (1992b). Dermatologic toxicity of chemotherapy. *Seminars in Oncology, 19,* 501–507.

DeVita, V.T., Carbone, P.P., Owens, A.H., Jr., Gold, G.I., Krant, M.J., & Edmonson, J. (1965). Clinical trials with 1, 3-bis (2-chloroethyl) -1-nitrosourea, NSC-409962. *Cancer Research, 25,* 1876–1881.

Dewys, W.D., Begg, C., Lavin, P.T., Band, P.R., Bennett, J.M., Bertino, J.R., Cohen, M.H., Douglass, H.O., Jr., Engstrom, P.F., Ezdinli, E.Z., Horton, J., Johnson, G.J., Moertel, C.G., Oken, M.M., Perlia, C., Rosenbaum, C., Silverstein, M.N., Skeel, R.T., Sponzo, R.W., & Tormey, D.C. (1980). Prognostic effect of weight loss prior to chemotherapy in cancer patients. Eastern Cooperative Oncology Group. *American Journal of Medicine, 69,* 491–497.

Dodd, M.J. (1991). *Managing the side effects of chemotherapy and radiation.* Norwalk, CT: Appleton & Lange.

Doroshow, J.H., Locker, G.Y., Gaasterland, D.E., Hubbard, S.P., Young, R.C., & Myers, C.E. (1981). Ocular irritation from high-dose methotrexate therapy: Pharmacokinetics of drug in the tear film. *Cancer, 48,* 2158–2162.

Dorr, R.T. (1990). Antidotes to vesicant chemotherapy extravasations. *Blood Reviews, 4*(1), 41–60.

Dorr, R.T. (1991). Chemoprotectants for cancer chemotherapy. *Seminars in Oncology, 18*(Suppl. 2), 48–58.

Dorr, R.T. (1994). Pharmacologic management of vesicant chemotherapy extravasations. In R.T. Dorr & D.D. Von Hoff (Eds.), *Cancer chemotherapy handbook* (2nd ed.). Norwalk, CT: Appleton & Lange.

Dorr, R.T., & Bool, K.L. (1995). Antidote studies of vinorelbine-induced skin ulceration in the mouse. *Cancer Chemotherapy Pharmacology, 36,* 290–292.

Dorr, R.T., Alberts, D.S., & Salmon, S.E. (1983). Cold protection from intradermal (ID) doxorubicin (DOX) ulceration in the mouse. *Proceedings of the Annual Meeting of the American Association of Cancer Residents, 24,* 255.

Dorr, R.T., Alberts, D.S., Einspahr, J., Mason-Liddil, N., & Soble, M. (1987). Experimental dacarbazine antitumor activity and skin toxicity in relation to light exposure and pharmachologic antidotes. *Cancer Treatment Reports, 71,* 267–272.

Dorr, R.T., Snead, K., & Liddil, J.D. (1996). Skin ulceration potential of paclitaxel in a mouse skin model in vivo. *Cancer, 78,* 152–156.

Dow, K.H. (1995). A review of late effects of cancer in women. *Seminars in Oncology Nursing, 11,* 128–136.

Dreizen, S., McCredie, K.B., Dicke, K.A., Zander, A.R., & Peters, L.J. (1979). Oral complications of bone marrow transplantation in adults with acute leukemia. *Postgraduate Medicine, 66*(5), 187–193.

Dudas, S. (1993). Altered body image and sexuality. In S.L. Groenwald, M.H. Frogge, M. Goodman, & C.H. Yarbro (Eds.), *Cancer nursing: Principles and practice* (3rd ed.) (pp. 719–733).

Dunne, C.F. (1989). Safe handling of antineoplastic agents: Self-learning module. *Cancer Nursing, 12,* 120–127.

Edgar, T.A., Lee, D.S., & Cousins, D.D. (1994). Experience with a national medication error reporting program. *American Journal of Hospital Pharmacy, 51,* 1335–1338.

Eilber, F.R., Morton, D.L., Eckardt, J., Grant, T., & Weisenburger, T. (1984). Limb salvage for skeletal and soft tissue sarcomas. *Cancer, 53,* 2579–2584.

Einhorn, M., & Davidson, I. (1964). Hepatotoxicity of mercaptopurine. *JAMA, 188,* 802–806.

Ersek, M., Scanlon, C., Glass, E., Ferrell, B.R., & Steeves, R. (1995). Priority ethical issues in oncology nursing: Current approaches and future directions. *Oncology Nursing Forum, 22,* 803–807.

Eskilsson, J., Albertsson, M., & Mercke, C. (1988). Adverse cardiac effects during induction chemotherapy treatment with cisplatin and 5-fluorouracil. *Radiotherapy and Oncology, 13*(1), 41–46.

Essayan, D.M., Kagey-Sobotka, A., Colarusso, P.J., Lichtenstein, L.M., Ozols, R.F., & King, E.D. (1996). Successful parenteral desensitization to paclitaxel. *Journal of Allergy and Clinical Immunology, 97*(1), 42–46.

Evans, S. (1991). Nursing measures in the prevention and treatment of renal cell damage associated with cisplatin administration. *Cancer Nursing, 14,* 91–97.

Fairley, K.F., Barrie, J.U., & Johnson, W. (1972). Sterility and testicular atrophy related to chemotherapy. *Lancet, 1,* 568–569.

Farber, S., Diamond, L.K., Mercer, R.D., Sylvester, R.F., & Wolff, J.A. (1948). Temporary remissions in acute leukemia in children produced by folic acid antagonist, 4-aminopteroly-glutamic acid (aminopterin). *New England Journal of Medicine, 238,* 787–793.

Ferrell, B.R., & Rivera, L.M. (1995). Ethical decision making in oncology: A case study approach. *Cancer Practice, 3,* 94–99.

Finley, R.S. (1992). Drug interactions in the oncology patient. *Seminars in Oncology Nursing, 8,* 95–101.

Fischer, D.S., Knobf, M.T., & Durivage, H.J. (1993). *The cancer chemotherapy handbook* (4th ed). St. Louis: Mosby.

Fisher, B., Costantino, J.P., Redmond, C.L., Fisher, E.R., Wickerham, D.L., & Cronin, W.M. (1994). Endometrial cancer in tamoxifen-treated breast cancer patients: Findings from the National Surgical Adjuvant Breast and Bowel Project (NSABP) B-14. *Journal of the National Cancer Institute, 86,* 527–537.

Fisher, B., Fisher, E., & Redmond, C. (1986). Ten-year results from the NSABP clinical trial evaluating the use of L-phenylalanine mustard (L-PAM) in the management of primary breast cancer. *Journal of Clinical Oncology, 4,* 929–941.

Fletcher, D.M. (1992). Unconventional cancer treatments: Professional, legal, and ethical issues. *Oncology Nursing Forum, 19,* 1351–1354.

Flynn, T.C., Harrist, T.J., Murphy, G.F., Loss, R.W., & Moschella, S.L. (1984). Neutrophilic eccrine hidradenitis: A distintive rash associated with cytarabine therapy and acute leukemia. *Journal of the American Academy of Dermatology, 11*(4, pt. 1), 584–590.

Forbes, J.F. (1992). Long-term effects of adjuvant chemotherapy in breast cancer. *Acta Oncologica, 31,* 243–250.

Frank-Stromborg, M., & Chamorro, T. (1996). Legal responsibilities of the nurse. In R. McCorkle, M. Grant, M. Frank-Stromborg, & S.B. Baird (Eds.), *Cancer nursing: A comprehensive textbook* (2nd ed.) (pp. 1388–1408). Philadelphia: Saunders.

Fraser, M.C., & Tucker, M.A. (1988). Late effects of cancer therapy: Chemotherapy-related malignancies. *Oncology Nursing Forum, 15,* 67–77.

Fraunfelder, F.T., & Meyer, S.M. (1987). Systemic reaction of ophthalmic drug prepartions. *Medical Toxicology Adverse Drug Experience, 2*(4), 287–293.

Friedman, L.S., & Isselbacher, K.J. (1994). Anorexia, nausea, vomiting, and indigestion. In J. Wilson (Ed.), *Harrison's principles of internal medicine* (13th ed.) (pp. 208–213). New York: McGraw-Hill.

Fuller, A.K. (1990). Platelet transfusion therapy for thrombocytopenia. *Seminars in Oncology Nursing, 6,* 123–128.

Gabrilove, J.L., Jakubowski, A., Scher, H., Sternberg, C., Wong, G., Grous, J., Yagoda, A., Fain, K., Moore, M., Clarkson, B., Oettgen, H., Alton, K., Welte, K., & Souza, L. (1988). Effect of granulocyte colony-stimulating factor on neutropenia and associated morbidity due to chemotherapy for transitional-cell cancer of the uroepithelium. *New England Journal of Medicine, 318,* 1414–1422.

Galassi, A. (1992). The next generation: New chemotherapy agents for the 1990s. *Seminars in Oncology Nursing, 8,* 83–94.

Gardner, S.F., Lazarus, H.M., Bednarczyk, E.M., Creger, R.J., Miraldi, F.D., Leisure, G., & Green, J.A. (1993). High-dose cyclophosphamide-induced myocardial damage during BMT: Assessment by positron emission tomography. *Bone Marrow Transplantation, 12*(2), 139–144.

Giacalone, S.B. (1997). Cancer clinical trials. In S.E. Otto (Ed.), *Oncology Nursing* (3rd ed.) (pp. 641-665). St. Louis: Mosby.

Gilman, A. (1963). The initial clinical trial of nitrogen mustard. *American Journal of Surgery, 105,* 574–578.

Gilman, A., & Philips, F.J. (1946). The biological actions of therapeutic applications of b-chloroethyl amines and sulfides. *Science, 103,* 409–415.

Ginsberg, S.J., & Comis, R.L. (1984). The pulmonary toxicity of antineoplastic agents. In M.C. Perry & J.W. Yarbro (Eds.), *Toxicity of chemotherapy* (pp. 227–268). New York: Grune & Stratton.

Glass, E. (1994, December). Coordinator's message: Ethics SIG survey results. *Ethics Special Interest Group Newsletter, 5*(2), 1, 4.

Glicksman, A.S., Pajak, T.F., Gottlieb, A., Nissen, N., Stutzman, L., & Cooper, M. (1982). Second malignant neoplasms in patients successfully treated for Hodgkin's disease: A cancer and leukemia group B study. *Cancer Treatment Reports, 66,* 1035–1044.

Gnarra, J., Lerman, M., Zbar, B., & Linehan, W.M. (1995). Genetics of renal-cell carcinoma and evidence for a critical role for von Hippel-Lindau in renal tumorigenesis. *Seminars in Oncology, 22,* 3–8.

Gomez, G.A., Aggarwal, K.K., & Han, T. (1982). Post-therapeutic acute malignant myeloproliferative syndrome and acute nonlymphocytic leukemia in non-Hodgkins lymphoma. *Cancer, 50,* 2285–2288.

Goodman, M., & Riley, M.B. (1997). Chemotherapy: Principles of administration. In S.L. Groenwald, M.H. Frogge, M. Goodman, & C.H. Yarbro (Eds.), *Cancer nursing: Principles and practice* (4th ed.) (pp. 317–384). Boston: Jones & Bartlett.

Grahan, G., & Johnson, J. (1990). Learning to cope and living with cancer: Learning-needs assessment in cancer patient education. *Scandinavian Journal of Caring Sciences, 4*(4), 173–181.

Graydon, J., Bubela, N., Irvine, D., & Vincent, L. (1995). Fatigue-reducing strategies used by patients receiving treatment for cancer. *Cancer Nursing, 18,* 23–28.

Green, L., & Donehower, R.C. (1984). Hepatic toxicity of low doses of mithramycin in hypercalcemia. *Cancer Treatment Reports, 68,* 1379–1381.

Greenberg, K., Sawicka, J., Eisenthal, S., & Ross, D. (1992). Fatigue syndrome due to localized radiation. *Journal of Pain and Symptom Management, 7,* 38–45.

Greene, M.H., Harris, E.L., Gershenson, D.M., Malkasian, G.D. Jr., Melton, L.J., III, Dembo, A.J., Bennett, J.M., Moloney, W.C., & Boice, J.D., Jr. (1986). Melphalan may be a more potent leukemogen than cyclophosphamide. *Annals of Internal Medicine, 105,* 360–367.

Gross, J. (1989). Cancer drug development. In L. Tenenbaum (Ed.), *Cancer chemotherapy: A reference guide* (pp. 99–109). Philadelphia: Saunders.

Guido, G.W. (1997). *Legal issues in nursing* (2nd ed.). Norwalk, CT: Appleton & Lange.

Gullo, S.M. (1988). Safe handling of antineoplasic drugs: Translating the recommendations into practice. *Oncology Nursing Forum, 15,* 595–601.

Guy, J.L., & Ingram, B.A. (1996). Medical oncology—The agents. In R. McCorkle, M. Grant, M. Frank-Stromborg, & S.B. Baird (Eds.), *Cancer nursing: A comprehensive textbook* (2nd ed.) (pp. 359–394). Philadelphia: Saunders.

Hancock, S.L., Tucker, M.A., & Hoppe, R.T. (1993). Mantle radiation therapy and MOPP. *Journal of the National Cancer Institute, 85,* 25–31.

Hardwick, N., & Murray, A. (1986). Inflammation of actinic keratosis induced by cytotoxic drugs [Letter to the editor]. *British Journal of Dermatology, 114,* 639–640.

Harrison, B. (1992). Safe handling of cytotoxic drugs: A review. In M. C. Perry (Ed.), *The chemotherapy source book* (pp. 799–832). Baltimore: Williams & Wilkins.

Harrist, T.J., Fine, J.D., Berman, R.S., Murphy, G.F., & Mihm, M.C., Jr. (1982). Neutrophilic eccrine hidradenitis: A distinctive type of neutophilic dermatosis associated with myelogenous leukemia and chemotherapy. *Archives of Dermatology, 118,* 263–266.

Harwood, K., & Govin, R. (1994). Short term vs. long term local cooling after doxorubicin (Dox) extravasation: An Eastern Cooperative Oncology Group (ECOG) study [Abstract]. *Program/Proceedings of the American Society of Clinical Oncology, 13,* 447.

Harwood, K.V., & Bachur, N. (1987). Evaluation of dimethyl sulfoxide and local cooling as antidotes for doxorubicin extravasation in a pig model. *Oncology Nursing Forum, 14*(1), 39–44.

Herrington, J.D., & Figueroa, J.A. (1997). Severe necrosis due to paclitaxel extravasation. *Pharmacology, 17,* 163–165.

Hesketh, P., & Gandara, D. (1991). Serotonin antagonists: A new class of antiemetic agents. *Journal of the National Cancer Institute, 83,* 613–620.

Hoagland, H.C. (1992). Hematologic complications of cancer chemotherapy. In M.C. Perry (Ed.), *The chemotherapy source book* (pp. 498–507). Baltimore: Williams & Wilkins.

Hoffman, D. (1980). The handling of antineoplastic drugs in a major cancer center. *Hospital Pharmacy, 15,* 302–304.

Hoffman, K.K., Weber, J., Samsa, G.P., & Rutala, W.A. (1992). Transparent polyurethane film as intravenous catheter dressing. *JAMA, 267,* 2072–2076.

Hogan, C. (1984). Vitamin E for stomatitis [Letter to the editor]. *Oncology Nursing Forum, 11*(2), 69.

Hoogstraten, B., Gottlieb, J.A., Caoili, E., Tucker, W.G., Talley, R.W., & Haut, A. (1973). CCNU (1, [2-chloroethyl]-3-cyclohexyl-1 nitrsourea, NSC-79037) in the treatment of cancer. Phase II study. *Cancer, 32,* 38–43.

Hopen, G., Mondino, B.J., Johnson, B.L., & Chervenick, P.A. (1981). Corneal toxicity with systemic cytarabine. *American Journal of Ophthalmology, 91,* 500–504.

Hoskins, K., Stopfer, J., Calzone, K., Merajver, S., Rebbeck, T., Garber, J., & Weber, B. (1995). Assessment and counseling for women with a family history of breast cancer, *JAMA, 273,* 577–585.

Hrozencik, S.P., & Connaughton, M.J. (1988). Cancer-associated hemolytic uremic syndrome. *Oncology Nursing Forum, 15,* 755–759.

Hubbard, S.M., & Seipp, C.A. (1985). Administration of cancer therapies: A practical guide for physicians and oncology nurses. In V.T. DeVita, S. Hellman, & S.A. Rosenberg (Eds.), *Cancer: Principles and practice of oncology* (2nd ed.) (pp. 2189–2222). Philadelphia: Lippincott.

Hydzik, C.A. (1990). Late effects of chemotherapy: Implications for patient management and rehabilitation. *Nursing Clinics of North America, 25,* 423–446.

Ignoffo, R.J., & Friedman, M.A. (1980). Therapy of local toxicities caused by extravasation of cancer chemotherapeutic drugs. *Cancer Treatment Reviews, 7*(1), 17–27.

Imperia, P.S., Lazarus, H.M., & Lass, J.H. (1989). Ocular complications of systemic cancer chemotherapy. *Survey of Ophthalmology, 34,* 209–230.

Irwin, M. (1987). Patients receiving biologic response modifiers: Overview of nursing care. *Oncology Nursing Forum, 14*(Suppl. 6), 32–37.

Jack, M.K., & Hicks, J.D. (1981). Ocular complications in high dose chemotherapy and marrow transplantation. *Annals of Ophthalmology, 13,* 709–711.

Jacobsen, P.B., Andrykowski, M.A., Redd, W.H., Die-Trill, M., Hakes, T.B., Kaufman, R.J., Currie, V.E., & Holland, J.C. (1988). Nonpharmacologic factors in the development of posttreatment nausea with adjuvant chemotherapy for breast cancer. *Cancer, 61,* 379–385.

Jackson, D. (1995). Latex allergy and anaphylaxis—What to do? *Journal of Intravenous Nursing, 18*(1), 33–52.

Jaffe, N., Paed, D., & Farber, S. (1973). Favorable response of metastatic osteogenic sarcoma to pulse high-dose methotrexate with citrovorum rescue and radiation therapy. *Cancer, 31,* 1367–1373.

Jaffe, N., Sullivan, M.P., Ried, H., Boren, H., Marshall, R., Meistrich, M., Maor, V., & da Cunha, M. (1988). Male reproductive function in long-term survivors of childhood cancer. *Medical and Pediatric Oncology, 16,* 241–247.

Jenkins, J., & Curt, G. (1996). Implementation of clinical trials. In R. McCorkle, M. Grant, M. Frank-Stromborg, & S.B. Baird (Eds.), *Cancer nursing: A comprehensive textbook* (2nd ed.) (pp. 470–484). Philadelphia: Saunders.

Jenkins, P.G., & Rieselbach, R.E. (1982). Acute renal failure: Diagnosis, clinical spectrum, and management. In R.E. Rieselbach & M.B. Garnick (Eds.), *Cancer and the kidney* (pp. 103–179). Philadelphia: Lea & Febiger.

Johnson, D.H., Greco, F.A., & Wolff, S.N. (1983). Etoposide-induced hepatic injury: A potential complication of high-dose therapy. *Cancer Treatment Reports, 67,* 1023–1024.

Johnson, T.M., Rapini, R.P., & Duvic, M. (1987). Inflammation of actinic keratosis from systemic chemotherapy. *Journal of the American Academy of Dermatology, 17*(2, pt. 1), 192–197.

Kaempfer, S.H., Wiley, F.M., Hoffman, D.J., & Rhodes, E.A. (1985). Fertility considerations and procreative alternatives in cancer care. *Seminars in Oncology Nursing, 1,* 25–34.

Kaiser, F.E. (1992). Sexual function and the older patient. *Oncology, 6*(Suppl. 2) 112–118.

Kaiser-Kupfer, M.I., & Lippman, M.E. (1978). Tamoxifen retinopathy. *Cancer Treatment Reports, 62,* 321–325.

Kantarjian, H.M., Keating, M.J., Walters, R.S., Smith, T., Cork, A., McCredie, K., & Fredireich, E. (1986). Therapy-related leukemia and myelodysplastic syndrome: Clinical, cytogenetic and prognostic features. *Journal of Clinical Oncology, 4,* 1748–1757.

Kaplan, R.S., & Wiernik, P.H. (1982). Neurotoxicity of antineoplastic agents. *Seminars in Oncology, 9,* 103 130.

Kaszyk, L.K. (1986). Cardiac toxicity associated with cancer therapy. *Oncology Nursing Forum, 13*(4), 81–88.

Katon, R.M. (1981). Complications of the upper gastrointestinal endoscopy in the gastrointestinal bleeder. *Digestive Diseases and Sciences, 26*(Suppl. 7), 47s–54s.

Kelly, B., & Mahon, S.M. (1988). Nursing care of the patient with multiple sclerosis. *Rehabilitation Nursing, 13,* 238–242.

Kende, G., Sirkin, S.R., Thomas, P.R., & Freeman, A.I. (1979). Blurring of vision. A previously undescribed complication of cyclophosphamide therapy. *Cancer, 44,* 69–71.

Kerker, B.J., & Hood, A.F. (1989). Chemotherapy-induced cutaneous reactions. *Seminars in Dermatology, 8*(3), 173–181.

Kodish, E., Stocking, C., Ratain, M.J., Kohrman, A., & Siegler, M. (1992). Ethical issues in phase I oncology research: A comparison of investigators and institutional review board chairpersons. *Journal of Clinical Oncology, 10,* 1810–1816.

Krebs, L.U. (1993). Sexual and reproductive dysfunction. In S.L. Groenwald, M.H. Frogge, M. Goodman, & C.H. Yarbro (Eds.), *Cancer nursing: Principles and practice* (3rd ed.) (pp. 696–718). Boston: Jones & Bartlett.

Kriesman, H., & Wolkove, N. (1992). Pulmonary toxicity of antineoplastic therapy. In M.C. Perry (Ed.), *The chemotherapy source book* (2nd ed.) (pp. 598–619). Baltimore: Williams & Wilkins.

Kroll, S.S., Koller, C.A., Kaled, S., & Dreizen, S. (1989). Chemotherapy-induced acral erythema: Desquamating lesions involving the hands and feet. *Annals of Plastic Surgery, 23,* 263–265.

Kumar, J. (1993). Epipodophyllotoxins and secondary leukaemia. *Lancet, 342,* 819–820.

Kupersmith, M.J., Frohman, L.P., Choi, I.S., Foo, S.H., Hiesinger, E., Berenstein, A., Wise, A., Carr, R.E., & Ransohoff, J. (1988). Visual system toxicity following intra-arterial chemotherapy. *Neurology, 38,* 284–289.

Labianca, R., Beretta, G., Clerici, M., Fraschini, P., & Luporini, G. (1982). Cardiac toxicity of 5-fluorouracil: A study of 1083 patients. *Tumori, 68,* 505–510.

Larson, D.K. (1985). What is the appropriate treatment of tissue extravasation by antitumor agents? *Plastic and Reconstructive Surgery, 75,* 397–405.

Lass, J.H., Lazarus, H.M., Reed, M.D., & Herzig, R.H. (1982). Topical corticosteroid therapy for corneal toxicity for systemically administered cytarabine. *American Journal of Ophthalmology, 94,* 617–621.

Laurie, S.W., Wilson, K.L., Kernahan, D.A., Bauer, B.S., & Vistnes, L.M. (1984). Intravenous extravasation injuries: The effectiveness of hyaluronidase in their treatment. *Annals of Plastic Surgery, 13*(3), 191–194.

Lavaud, F., Prevost, A., Cossart, C., Guerin, L., Bernard, J., & Kochman, S. (1995). Allergy to latex, avocado, pear, and banana: Evidence for a 30 kd antigen in immunoblotting. *The Journal of Allergy and Clinical Imunology, 95,* 557–564.

LeBeau, M.M., Albain, K.S., Larson, R.A., Vardiman, J., Dvais, E., Blough, R., Golomb, H., & Rowley, J. (1986). Clinical and cytogenetic correlations in 63 patients with therapy-related myelodysplastic syndromes and acute nonlymphocytic leukemia: Further evidence for characteristic abnormalities of chromosome nos. 5 and 7. *Journal of Clinical Oncology, 4,* 325–345.

Lindower, P., & Skorton, D. (1992). The cardiovascular system and anticancer therapy. In J.O. Armitage & K.H. Antman (Eds.), *High dose cancer therapy: Pharmacology, hematopoietins, stem cells* (pp. 505–517). Baltimore: Williams & Wilkins.

Lopez, M. (1992). Central venous access for chemotherapy. In M.C. Perry (Ed.), *The chemotherapy source book* (pp. 780–798). Baltimore: Williams & Wilkins.

Lydon, J. (1980). Assessment of renal function in the patient receiving chemotherapy. *Cancer Nursing, 12,* 133–143.

Lydon, J. (1986). Nephrotoxicity of cancer treatment. *Oncology Nursing Forum, 13*(2), 68–77.

Macdonald, D.R. (1991). Neurologic complications of chemotherapy. *Neurologic Clinics, 9,* 955–967.

MacVicar, M., Winningham, M., & Nickel, J. (1989). Effects of aerobic interval training on cancer patients' functional capacity. *Nursing Research, 38,* 348–351.

Malkin, D., Jolly, K.W., Barbier, N., Look, T., Friend, S., Gebhart, M., Andersen, T., Borresen, A., Li, F., Garber, J., & Strong, L. (1992). Germline mutations of the p53 tumor suppressor gene in children and young adults with second malignant neoplasms. *New England Journal of Medicine, 326,* 1309–1315.

Marcial, V.A., Pajak, T.F., Kramer, S., Davis, L.W., Steta, J., Laramore, G.E., Jacobs, J.R., Al-Sarraf, M., & Brady, L.W. (1988). Radiation Therapy Oncology Group (RTOG) studies in head and neck cancer. *Seminars in Oncology, 15,* 39–60.

Margileth, D.A., Poplack, D.G., Pizzo, P.A., & Leventhal, B.G. (1977). Blindness during remission in two patients with acute lymphoblastic leukemia: A possible complication of multimodality therapy. *Cancer, 39,* 58–61.

Marsee, V. (1994). Ethical dilemmas in the delivery of intensive care to critically ill oncology patients. *Seminars in Oncology Nursing, 10,* 156–164.

Martin-Jimenez, M., Diaz-Rubio, E., Larriba, J.L., & Sangra, L. (1986). Failure of high-dose tocopherol to prevent alopecia induced by doxorubicin. *New England Journal of Medicine, 315,* 894–895.

Maxson, J.H., & Wolk, J.E. (1998). Principles of preparation, administration, and disposal of antineoplastic agents. In J.K. Itano & K.N. Taoka (Eds.), *Core curriculum for oncology nursing* (3rd ed.) (pp. 157–661). Philadelphia: Saunders.

Mayo, D.J., & Pearson, D.C. (1995). Chemotherapy extravasation: A consequence of fibrin sheath formation around venous access devices. *Oncology Nursing Forum, 22,* 675–680.

McCabe, M.S. (1993). The ethical context of healthcare reform. *Oncology Nursing Forum, 20*(Suppl. 10), 35–43.

McDonald, G.B., & Tirumali, N. (1984). Intestinal and liver toxicity of antineoplastic drugs. *Western Journal of Medicine, 140,* 250–259.

McDonald, G.B., Hinds, M., Fisher L., & Schoch, H.G. (1993). Veno occlusive disease of the liver and multiorgan failure after bone marrow transplantation: A cohort study of 355 patients. *Annals of Internal Medicine, 118,* 255–267.

McGrath, P. (1995). It's ok to say no! A discussion of ethical issues arising from informed consent to chemotherapy. *Cancer Nursing, 18,* 97–103.

Mead Johnson Oncology Products. (1994). Taxol (paclitaxel) [Package insert]. Princeton, NJ: Bristol-Myers Squibb.

Medication administration & I.V. therapy manual. (1993). Springhouse, PA: Springhouse Corporation.

Meehan, J., & Johnson, B. (1992). The neurotoxicity of antineoplastic agents. *Current Issues in Cancer Nursing Practice Updates, 1*(8), 1–11.

Meeske, K., & Ruccione, K.S. (1987). Cancer chemotherapy in children: Nursing issues and approaches. *Seminars in Oncology Nursing, 3,* 118–127.

Miki, Y., Swensen, J., Shattuck-Eidens, D., Futreal, P.A., Harshman, K., Tavtigian, S., Liu, Q., Cochran, C., Bennett, L.M., Ding, W., Bell, R., Rosenthal, J., Hussey, C., Tran, T., McClure, M., Frye, C., Hattier, T., Phelps, R. Haugen-Strano, A., Katcher, H., Yakumo, K., Gholami, Z., Shaffer, D., Stone, S., Bayer, S., Wray, C., Bogden, R., Dayananth, P., Ward, J., Tonin, P., Narod, S., Bristow, P., Norris, F., Helvering, L., Morrison, P., Rosteck, P., Lai, M., Barrett, J., Lewis, C., Neuhausen, S., Cannon-Albright, L., Goldgar, D., Wiseman, R., Kamb, A., & Skolnick, M. (1994). A strong candidate for the breast and ovarian cancer susceptibility gene *BRCA1. Science, 266,* 66–71.

Mills, B.A., & Roberts, R.W. (1979). Cyclophosphamide-induced cardio-myopathy: A report of two cases and review of the English literature. *Cancer, 43,* 2223–2226.

Mitchell, E.P., & Schein, P.S. (1982). Gastrointestinal toxicity of chemotherapeutic agents. *Seminars in Oncology, 9,* 52–64.

Mock, V., Burke, M.B., Sheehan, P., Creator, E., Winningham, M., McKinney-Tedder, S., Schwager, L.P., & Liebman, M. (1994). A nursing rehabilitation program for women with breast cancer receiving adjuvant chemotherapy. *Oncology Nursing Forum, 21,* 899–907.

Montrose, P. (1987). Extravasation management. *Seminars in Oncology Nursing, 3,* 128–132.

Moscow, J., & Cowan, K. (1988). Multidrug resistance. *Journal of the National Cancer Institute, 80,* 14–20.

Myerowitz, R.L., Sartiano, G.P., & Cavallo, T. (1976). Nephrotoxic and cytoproliferative effects of streptozotocin. *Cancer, 38,* 1550–1555.

Nail, L. (1997). Fatigue. In S.L. Groenwald, M.H. Frogge, M. Goodman, & C.H. Yarbro (Eds.), *Cancer nursing: Principles and practice* (4th ed.) (pp. 640-654). Boston: Jones & Bartlett.

Nail, L., & King, K. (1987). Fatigue. *Seminars in Oncology Nursing, 3,* 257–262.

National Cancer Institute. (1998). *Taking part in clinical trials: What cancer patients need to know* (NIH Publication No. 98-4250). Bethesda, MD: Author.

Nieweg, R., Van Tinteren, H., Poelhuis, E.K., & Abraham-Inpijn, L. (1992). Nursing care for oral complications associated with chemotherapy: A survey among members of the Dutch nursing society. *Cancer Nursing 15,* 313–321.

Norton, L. (1992) The Norton-Simon Hypothesis. In M.C. Perry (Ed.), *The chemotherapy source book* (pp. 36–53). Baltimore: Williams & Wilkins.

O'Rourke, M., Crawford, J., Schiller, J., Laufman, L., Yanovich, S., Ozer, H., Langeben, A., Barlogie, B., Koletsky, A., Clamon, G., Purvis, J., Tuttle, R., & Hohneker, J. (1993). Survival advantage for patients with stage IV non-small cell lung cancer treated with single agent navelbine in a randomized controlled trial [Abstract #1148]. *Proceedings of the American Society of Clinical Oncology, 12.*

Obama, M., Cangir, A., & van Eys, J. (1983). Nutritional status and anthracycline cardiotoxicity in children. *Southern Medical Journal, 76,* 577–578.

Occupational Safety and Health Administration. (1995). *Controlling occupational exposure to hazardous drugs* (OSHA Instruction CPL 2-2.20B). Washington, DC: Author.

Ofstehage, J.C., & Magilvy, K. (1986). Oral health and aging. *Geriatric Nursing, 7,* 238–241.

Olver, I.N., Aisner, J., Hament, A., Buchanan, L., Bishop, J.F., & Kaplan, R.S. (1988). A prospective study of topical dimethyl sulfoxide for treating anthracycline extravasation. *Journal of Clinical Oncology, 6,* 1732–1735.

Oncology Nursing Society. (1997). *Statement on the scope and standards of advanced practice in oncology nursing.* Pittsburgh: Oncology Nursing Press, Inc.

Ortho Biotech Corporation. (1994). Procrit (epoetin alfa) [Package insert]. Raritan, NJ: Author.

Oster, W., Herrmann, F., Cicco, A., Gamm, H., Zeile, G., Brune, T., Lindemann, A., Schulz, G., & Mertelsmann, R. (1990). Erythropoietin prevents chemotherapy-induced anemia: Case report. *Blood, 60*(2), 88–92.

Ostrow, S., Hahn, D., Wiernik, P.H., Richards, R.D. (1978). Ophthalmologic toxicity after cis-dichlorodiammineplatinum (II) therapy. *Cancer Treatment Reports, 62,* 591–594.

Otto, S. (Ed.). (1997). *Oncology nursing.* St. Louis: Mosby.

Ozols, R.F., Ostchega, Y., Curt, G., & Young, R. (1987). High-dose carboplatin in refractory ovarian cancer patients. *Journal of Clinical Oncology, 5,* 197–201.

Patterson, W.P., & Reams, G.P. (1992). Renal and electrolyte abnormalities due to chemotherapy. In M.C. Perry (Ed.), *The chemotherapy source book* (pp. 648–665). Baltimore: Williams & Wilkins.

Pedersen-Bjergaard, J., Philip, P., Larsen, S., Jensen, G., & Byrsting, K. (1990). Chromosome aberrations and prognostic factors in therapy related myelodysplasia and acute nonlymphocytic leukemia. *Blood, 76,* 1083–1091.

Perez, E. (1995). Review of the preclinical pharmacology and comparative efficacy of 5-hydroxytryptamine-3 receptor antagonists for chemotherapy-induced emesis. *Journal of Clinical Oncology, 13,* 1036–1043.

Perez, J.E., Macchiavelli, M., Leone, B.A., Romero, A., Rabinovich, M.G., Goldar, D., & Vallejo, C. (1986). High-dose alpha-tocopherol as a preventive of doxorubicin-induced alopecia. *Cancer Treatment Reports, 70,* 1213–1214.

Perry, M.C. (1992). Hepatotoxicity of chemotherapeutic agents. In M.C. Perry (Ed.), *The chemotherapy source book* (pp. 635–647). Baltimore: Williams & Wilkins.

Pervan, V. (1990). Current concepts in emesis control: Practical aspects of dealing with cancer therapy-induced nausea and vomiting. *Seminars in Oncology Nursing, 6*(Suppl. 1) 3–5.

Peterson, D.E., & Schubert, M.M. (1992). Oral toxicity. In M.C. Perry (Ed.), *The chemotherapy source book* (pp. 508–530). Baltimore: Williams & Wilkins.

Petros, W.P., & Peters, W.P. (1993). Hematopoietic colony-stimulating factors and dose intensity. *Seminars in Oncology, 20,* 94–99.

Pharmacia and Upjohn, Inc. (1996). Zinecard (dexrazoxane) [Package insert]. Kalamazoo, MI: Author.

Phillips, T.L., & Fu, K.K. (1977). Acute and late effects of multimodal therapy on normal tissues. *Cancer, 40*(Suppl. 1), 489–494.

Pickett, M. (1991). Determinants of anticipatory nausea and anticipatory vomiting in adults receiving cancer chemotherapy. *Cancer Nursing, 14,* 334–343.

Piper, B. (1991). Alterations in energy: The sensation of fatigue. In S.B. Baird, R. McCorkle, & M. Grant (Eds.), *Cancer nursing: A comprehensive textbook.* (pp. 894–908). Philadelphia: Saunders.

Piper, B., Dibble, S., Dodd, M., Weiss, M., Slaugher, R. & Paul, S. (1998). The revised Piper Fatigue Scale: Psychometric evaluation in women with breast cancer. *Oncology Nursing Forum, 25,* 677–684.

Pisters, K.W., & Kris, M.G. (1992). Management of nausea and vomiting caused by anticancer drugs: State of the art. *Oncology, 6*(Suppl. 2), 99–104.

Podurgiel, B.J., McGill, D.B., Luwig, J., Taylor, W.F., & Muller, S.A. (1973). Liver injury associated with methotrexate therapy for psoriasis. *Mayo Clinic Proceedings, 48*(1), 787–792.

Pollera, C.F., Ameglio, F., Nardi, M., Vitelli, G., & Marolla, P. (1987). Cisplatin-induced hepatic toxicity [Letter to the editor]. *Journal of Clinical Oncology, 5,* 318–319.

Portenoy, R.K. (1987). Constipation in the cancer patient: Causes and management. *Medical Clinics of North America, 71*(2), 303–312.

Pottage, A., Holt, S., Ludgate, S., & Langlands, A.O. (1978). Fluorouracil cardiotoxicity. *British Medical Journal, 1*(6112), 547.

Raymond, J.R. (1984). Nephrotoxicities and antineoplastic and immunosuppressive agents. *Current Problems in Cancer, 8*(16), 1–32.

Redd, W.H., Burish, T.G., & Andrykowski, M.A. (1985). Aversive conditioning and cancer chemotherapy. In T.G. Burish, S.M. Levy, & B.E. Meyerowitz (Eds.), *Cancer, nutrition, and eating behavior: A biobehavioral perspective* (pp. 117–132). Hillsdale, NJ: Lawrence Erlbaum Associates, Inc.

Richards, C., & Wujcik, D. (1992). Cutaneous toxicity associated with high-dose cytosine arabinoside. *Oncology Nursing Forum, 19,* 1191–1195.

Rodu, B., Russell, C.M., & Ray, K.L. (1988). Treatment of oral ulcers with hydroxypropyl cellulose film. *Compendium, 9,* 420–422.

Rousseau, L., Dupont, A., Labrie, F., & Couture, M. (1988). Sexuality changes in prostate cancer patients receiving antihormonal therapy combining the antiandrogen flutamide with medical (LHRH agonist) or surgical castration. *Archives of Sexual Behavior, 17,* 87–98.

REFERENCES

Rowinsky, E., McGuire, W., Guarnieri, T., Fisherman, J., Christian, M., & Donehower, R. (1991). Cardiac disturbances during the administration of Taxol. *Journal of Clinical Oncology, 9,* 1704–1712.

Rowinsky, E., Onetto, N., Canetta, R., & Arbuck, S. (1992). Taxol: The first of the taxanes, an important new class of antitumor agents. *Seminars in Oncology, 19,* 646–662.

Rudolph, R., & Larson, D.L. (1987). Etiology and treatment of chemotherapeutic agent extravasation injuries: A review. *Journal of Clinical Oncology, 5,* 1116–1126.

Rutqvist, L.E., Johansson, H., Signomklao, T., Johansson, U., Fornander, T., & Wilking, N. (1995). Adjuvant tamoxifen therapy for early stage breast cancer and second primary malignancies. *Journal of the National Cancer Institute, 87,* 645–651.

Sadoff, L. (1979). Nephrotoxicity of streptozotocin (NSC85998). *Cancer Chemotherapy Reports, 54,* 457–459.

Sahlin, K. (1992). Metabolic factors in fatigue. *Sports Medicine, 13*(2), 99–107.

Sandler, S.G., Tobin, W., & Henderson, E.S. (1969). Vincristine induced neuropathy: A clinical study of fifty leukemic patients. *Neurology, 19,* 367–374.

Sansivero, G.E., & Murray, S.A. (1989). Safe management of chemotherapy at home. *Oncology Nursing Forum, 16,* 711–713.

Scanlon, C. (1994). Survey yields significant results. *American Nurses Association Center for Ethics and Human Rights Communiqué, 3*(3), 1–3.

Schilsky, R.L., & Erlichman, C. (1982). Late complications of chemotherapy: Infertility and carcinogenesis. In B. Chabner (Ed.), *Pharmacologic principles of cancer treatment* (pp. 109–128). Philadelphia: Saunders.

Schilsky, R.L., Lewis, B.J., & Sherins, R.J. (1980). Gonadal dysfunction in patients receiving chemotherapy for cancer. *Annals of Internal Medicine, 93,* 109–114.

Schlang, H.A., & Curtin, R. (1977). Inflammation of malignant skin involvement with fluorouracil [Letter to the editor]. *JAMA, 238,* 1722.

Schulmeister, L. (1987). Litigation involving oncology nurses. *Oncology Nursing Forum,14*(2), 25–28.

Schulmeister, L. (1993). Documentation issues in oncology nursing. *Current Issues in Cancer Nursing Practice Updates, 1*(9), 1–8.

Schulmeister, L. (1997). Preventing chemotherapy dose and schedule errors. *Clinical Journal of Oncology Nursing, 1,* 79–85.

Schulmeister, L. (1998). Negligence and malpractice in oncology nursing. *Clinical Journal of Oncology Nursing, 2,* 25–26.

Scofield, R.P., Liebman, M.C., & Popkin, J.D. (1991). Multimodal therapy. In S.B. Baird, R. McCorkle, & M. Grant (Eds.), *Cancer nursing: A comprehensive textbook* (pp. 344–354). Philadelphia: Saunders.

Scuderi, N., & Onesti, M.G. (1994). Antitumor agents: Extravasation, managment and surgical treatment. *Annals of Plastic Surgery, 32*(1), 39–44.

Selby, P., Brada, M., Horwich, A., Wiltshaw, E., McElwain, T.J., & Lindsay, K.S. (1988). Semen cryopreservation for patients surviving malignant disease. Implications for proposed legislation. *Lancet, 2,* 1197.

Shaffer, S. (1994). Protective mechanisms. In S.E. Otto (Ed.), *Oncology nursing* (2nd ed.) (pp. 698–719). St. Louis: Mosby.

Shall, L., Lucus, G.S., Whittaker, J.A., & Holt, P.J. (1988). Painful red hands: A side-effect of leukemia therapy. *British Journal of Dermatology, 119,* 249–253.

Shenkenberg, T.D., & Von Hoff, D.D. (1986). Mitoxantrone: A new anticancer drug with significant clinical activity. *Annals of Internal Medicine, 105*(1), 67–81.

Shepherd, J.D., Pringle, L.E., Barnett, M.J., Klingemann, H.G., Reece, D.E., & Phillips, G.L. (1991). Mesna versus hyperhydration for the prevention of cyclophosphamide-induced hemorrhagic cystitis in bone marrow transplantation. *Journal of Clinical Oncology, 9,* 2016–2020.

Skalla, K., & Lacasse, C. (1992). Patient education for fatigue. *Oncology Nursing Forum, 19,* 1537–1541.

Skeel, R.T. (Ed.). (1991). *Handbook of cancer chemotherapy* (3rd ed.). Boston: Little, Brown, & Co.

Slichenmyer, W.J., Rowinsky, E.K., Donehower, R.C., & Kaufmann, S.H. (1993). The current status of camptothecin analogues as antitumor agents. *Journal of the National Cancer Institute, 85,* 271–291.

Smith, D.S., & Charmarro, T.P. (1978). Nursing care of patients undergoing combination chemotherapy and radiotherapy. *Cancer Nursing, 1,* 129–134.

Smith, M.A., Rubinstein, L., & Ungerleider, R.S. (1994). Therapy-related acute myeloid leukemia following treatment with epipodophyllotoxins: Estimating the risks. *Medical and Pediatric Oncology, 23,* 86–98.

Smith, S.P. (1987). *Handling, storage, and disposal of antineoplastic drugs: Policy and procedure.* Hartford, CT: Mt. Sinai Hospital.

Soble, M.J., Dorr, R.T., Plezia, P., & Breckenridge, S. (1987). Dose-dependent skin ulcers in mice treated with DNA binding antitumor antibiotics. *Cancer Chemotherapy & Pharmacology, 20*(1), 33–36.

Solomon, M.A. (1986). Oral sucralfate suspension for mucositis [Letter to the editor]. *New England Journal of Medicine, 315,* 459–460.

Spaeth, G.L., & Von Sallmann, L. (1966). Corticosteroids and cataracts. *International Ophthalmology Clinics, 6,* 915–928.

Speyer, J., Green, M., Dramer, E., Rey, M., Sanger, J., Ward, C., Dubin, N., Ferrans, V., Stegy, P., Zellenuch-Jacqcotta, A., Wernz, J., Felt, F., Slater, W., & Muggia, F. (1988). Protective effect of the bispiperazinedione ICRF-187 against doxorubicin-induced cardiac toxicity in women with advanced breast cancer. *New England Journal of Medicine, 319,* 745–752.

Speyer, J.L., Green, M.D., Zeleniuch-Jacquotte, A., Wernz, J.C., Rey, M., Sanger, J., Kramer, E., Ferrans, V., Hochester, H., Meyers, M., Blum, R.H., Feit, F., Attubato, M., Burrows, W., & Muggia, F.M. (1992). ICRF-187 permits longer treatment with doxorubicin in women with breast cancer. *Journal of Clinical Oncology, 10,* 117–127.

St. Germain, B., Houlihan, N., & D'Amato, S. (1994). Dimethyl sulfoxide therapy in the treatment of vesicant extravasation: Two case presentations. *Journal of Intravenous Nursing, 17,* 261–266.

Stehling, L., Luban, N., Anderson, K., Sayers, M., Attar, S., Leitman, S., Gould, S., Kruskall, M., Goodnough, L., & Hines, D. (1994). Guidelines for blood utilization review. *Transfusion, 34,* 438–448.

Stillwell, T.J., & Benson, R.C., Jr. (1988). Cyclophosphamide-induced hemorrhagic cystitis: A review of 100 patients. *Cancer, 61,* 451–457.

Stott, H., Fox, W., Girling, D.J., Stephens, R.J., & Galton, D.A. (1977). Acute leukemia after busulphan. *British Medical Journal, 2*(6101), 1513–1517.

Sweet, V., Servy, E.J., & Karow, A.M. (1996). Reproductive issues for men with cancer: Technology and nursing management. *Oncology Nursing Forum, 23,* 51–58.

Symann, M. (1991). Hematopoietic growth factors as supportive therapy for cancer and chemotherapy-induced conditions. *Current Opinion in Oncology, 3,* 648–655.

Tabak, N. (1995). Decision making in consenting to experimental cancer therapy. *Cancer Nursing, 18*(2), 89–96.

Tchekmedyian, N.S. (1993). *Managing cancer cachexia.* Princeton, NJ: Bristol-Myers Squibb.

Tenenbaum, L. (1989). *Cancer chemotherapy: A reference guide.* Philadelphia: Saunders.

Thelan, L.A., Davie, J.K., Urden, L.D., & Lough, M.E. (1994). *Critical care nursing: Diagnosis and management* (2nd ed.). St. Louis: Mosby.

Thomas, C. (Ed.). (1997). *Taber's cyclopedic medical dictionary* (18th ed.). Philadelphia: F.A. Davis.

Thomasma, D.C. (1997). Ethical issues in cancer nursing practice. In S.L. Groenwald, M.H. Frogge, M. Goodman, & C.H. Yarbro (Eds.), *Cancer nursing: Principles and practice* (4th ed.) (pp. 1608–1624). Boston: Jones & Bartlett.

Thurman, W.G., Bloedow, C., Howe, C.D., Levin, W.C., Davis, P., Lane, M., Sullivan, M.P., & Griffith, K.M. (1963). A phase I study of hydoxyurea. *Cancer Chemotherapy Reports, 29,* 103–107.

Tonato, M., Aapro, M., Andrews, P., Boyce, M.J., Del Favero, A., Gandara, D., Gralla, R.J., Grunberg, S., Joss, R., Kris, R., Martin, M., & Roila, F. (1993). Supportive therapy: Challenges for the '90s—Perspectives in antiemetic therapy. *European Journal of Cancer, 29A*(Suppl. 1), S42–S51.

Tortorice, P.V. (1997). Chemotherapy: Principles of therapy. In S.L. Growenwald, M.H. Frogge, M. Goodman, & C.H. Yarbro (Eds.), *Cancer nursing: Principles and practice* (4th ed.) (pp. 283–316). Boston: Jones & Bartlett.

Travis, L.B., Curtis, R., Glimelius, B., Holowaty, E., Van Leeuwen, F., Lynch, C., Hagenbeek, A., Stovall, M., Banks, P., Adami, J., Gospodarowicz, M., Wacholder, S., Inskip, P., Tucker, M., & Boice, J. (1995). Bladder and kidney cancer following cyclophosphamide therapy for non-Hodgkin's lymphoma. *Journal of the National Cancer Institute, 87,* 524–530.

Tsavaris, N., Caragiauris, P., & Kosmidis, P. (1988). Reduction of oral toxicity of 5-fluorouracil by allopurinol mouthwashes. *European Journal of Surgical Oncology, 14,* 405–406.

Tucker, M.A., Coleman, C.N., Cox, R.S., Varghese, A., & Rosenberg, S.A. (1988). Risk of second cancers after treatment for Hodgkin's disease. *New England Journal of Medicine, 318,* 76–81.

Twycross, R.G., & Lack, S.A. (1986). *Control of alimentary symptoms in far advanced cancer.* New York: Churchill Livingstone.

Van Barneveld, P.W., van der Mark, T.W., Sleijfer, D.T., Mulder, N.H., Koops, H.S., Sluiter, H.J., & Peset, R. (1984). Predictive factors for bleomycin-induced pneumonitis. *American Review of Respiratory Disease, 130,* 1078–1081.

Van Leeuwen, F.E., Klokman, W.J., Hagenbeek, A., Noyon, R., van den Belt-Dusebout, A.W., van Kerkhoff, E., van Heerde, P., & Somers, R. (1994). Second cancer risk following Hodgkin's disease: A 20-year follow-up study. *Journal of Clinical Oncology, 12,* 312–325.

Vander, J.K., Kincaid, M.C., Hegarty, T.J., Page, M., Averill, D., Junck, L., & Greenberg, H.S. (1990). The ocular effects of intracarotid bromodeoryuridine and radiation therapy in the treatment of malignant glioma. *Ophthalmology, 97,* 352–357.

Vizel, M., & Oster, M.W. (1982). Ocular side effects of cancer chemotherapy. *Cancer, 49,* 1999–2002.

Vogelzang, N.J. (1991). Nephrotoxicity from chemotherapy: Prevention and management. *Oncology, 5*(10), 97–102.

Von Hoff, D.D., Layard, M.W., Basa, P., Davis, H.L., Jr., Von Hoff, A.L., Rozencweig, M., & Muggia, F.M. (1979). Risk factors for doxorubicin-induced congestive heart failure. *Annals of Internal Medicine, 91,* 710–717.

Von Hoff, D.D., Rosenzweig, M., Layard, M., Slavik, M., & Muggia, F.M. (1977). Daunomycin-induced cardiotoxicity in children and adults: A review of 110 cases. *American Journal of Medicine, 62,* 200–208.

Vukelja, S.J., Lombardo, F.A., James, W.D., & Weiss, R.B. (1989). Pyridoxine for the palmar-plantar erythrodysesthesia syndrome [Letter to the editor] [published erratum appears in *Annals of Internal Medicine*, 1990, *112,* 151]. *Annals of Internal Medicine, 111,* 688–689.

Wahlquist, G. (1985). Mobility. In B.L. Johnson & J. Gross (Eds.), *Handbook of oncology nursing* (pp. 303–320). New York: John Wiley & Sons.

Wall, R.L., & Clausen, K.P. (1975). Carcinoma of the urinary bladder in patients receiving cyclophosphamide. *New England Journal of Medicine, 293,* 271–273.

Walsh, S., Begg, C., & Carbine, P. (1989). Cancer chemotherapy in the elderly. *Seminars in Oncology, 16,* 66–75.

Weber, B., Vogel, C., Jones, S., Harvey, H., Hutchins, L., Purvis, J., & Hohneker, J. (1993). A U.S. multicenter phase II trial of navelbine in advanced breast cancer [Abstract #46]. *Proceedings of the American Society of Clinical Oncology, 12,* 61.

Weiss, R.B. (1992a). Hypersensitivity reactions. In M.C. Perry (Ed.), *The chemotherapy source book* (pp. 553–569). Baltimore: Williams & Wilkins.

Weiss, R.B. (1992b). Hypersensitivity reactions. *Seminars in Oncology, 19,* 458–477.

Welch, D., & Lewis, K. (1980). Alopecia and chemotherapy . . . the ice turban. *American Journal of Nursing, 80,* 903–905.

Welch, J., & Silveira, J.M. (1997). *Safe handling of cytotoxic drugs: An independent study module* (2nd ed.). Pittsburgh: Oncology Nursing Press, Inc., a subsidiary of the Oncology Nursing Society.

Wickham, R. (1986). Pulmonary toxicity secondary to cancer treatment. *Oncology Nursing Forum, 13*(5), 69–76.

Wickham, R. (1989). Managing chemotherapy-related nausea and vomiting: The state of the art. *Oncology Nursing Forum, 16,* 563–574.

Wickham, R. (1990). Advances in venous access devices and nursing management strategies. *Nursing Clinics of North America, 25,* 345–364.

Wickham, R., Purl, S., & Welker, D. (1992). Long term central venous catheters: Issues for care. *Seminars in Oncology Nursing, 8,* 133–147.

Wilding, G., Caruso, R., Lawrence, T.S., Ostchega, Y., Ballintine, E.J., Young, R.C., & Ozols, R.F. (1985). Retinal toxicity after high-dose cisplatin therapy. *Journal of Clinical Oncology, 3,* 1683–1689.

Wille, J.C., Blusse Van Oud Albas, A.F., & Thewessen, E.A. (1993). A comparison of two transparent film-type dressings in central venous therapy. *Journal of Hospital Infection, 23,* 113–121.

Winningham, M.L. (1991). Walking program for people with cancer: Getting started. *Cancer Nursing, 14,* 270–276.

Winningham, M.L. (1992). How exercise mitigates fatigue: Implications for people receiving cancer therapy. In R.M. Carroll-Johnson (Ed.), *The Biotherapy of Cancer—V* (pp. 16–21). Pittsburgh: Oncology Nursing Press, Inc.

Winningham, M.L., & MacVicar, M.G. (1988). The effect of aerobic exercise on patient reports of nausea. *Oncology Nursing Forum, 15,* 447–450.

Winningham, M.L., Nail, L., Burke, M.B., Brophy, L., Cimprich, B., Jones, L., Pickard-Holley, S., Rhodes, V., St. Pierre, B., Beck, S., Glass, E., Mock, V., Mooney, K., & Piper, B. (1994). Fatigue and the cancer experience: The state of the knowledge. *Oncology Nursing Forum, 21,* 23–36.

Witman, G., Cadman, E., & Chen, M. (1981). Misuse of scalp hypothermia. *Cancer Treatment Reports, 65,* 507–508.

Wood, L.S., & Gullo, S.M. (1993). IV vesicants: How to avoid extravasation *American Journal of Nursing, 93*(4), 42–46.

Wrenn, K. (1989). Fecal impaction. *New England Journal of Medicine, 321,* 658–662.

Wroblewski, S.S., & Wroblewski, S.H. (1981). Caring for the patient with chemotherapy-induced thrombocytopenia. *American Journal of Nursing, 81,* 746–749.

Wujcik, D., & Downs, S. (1992). Bone marrow transplantation. *Critical Care Nursing Clinics of North America, 4*(1), 149–166.

Yarbro J. (1992). The scientific basis of cancer chemotherapy. In M.C. Perry (Ed.), *The chemotherapy source book* (pp. 2–14). Baltimore: Williams & Wilkins.

Zalupski, M., & Baker, L.H. (1988). Ifosfamide. *Journal of the National Cancer Institute, 80,* 556–566.

Zubrod, C.G. (1984). Origins and development of chemotherapy research at the National Cancer Institute. *Cancer Treatment Reports, 68,* 9–19.

Adverse Event	Grade				
	0	1	2	3	4

Appendix 1. National Cancer Institute Common Toxicity Criteria (CTC)

ALLERGY/IMMUNOLOGY

Adverse Event	0	1	2	3	4
Allergic reaction/ hypersensitivity (including drug fever)	none	transient rash, drug fever < 38°C (< 100.4°F)	urticaria, drug fever ≥ 38°C (≥ 100.4°F), and/ or asymptomatic bronchospasm	symptomatic bronchospasm, requiring parenteral medication(s), with or without urticaria; allergy-related edema/ angioedema	anaphylaxis

Note: Isolated urticaria, in the absence of other manifestations of an allergic or hypersensitivity reaction, is graded in the DERMATOLOGY/ SKIN category.

Adverse Event	0	1	2	3	4
Allergic rhinitis (including sneezing, nasal stuffiness, postnasal drip)	none	mild, not requiring treatment	moderate, requiring treatment	-	-
Autoimmune reaction	none	serologic or other evidence of autoim-mune reaction but patient is asymptom-atic (e.g., vitiligo), all organ function is normal, and no treatment is required	evidence of autoim-mune reaction involving a non-essential organ or function (e.g., hypothyroidism), requiring treatment other than immuno-suppressive drugs	reversible autoimmune reaction involving function of a major organ or other toxicity (e.g., transient colitis or anemia), requiring short-term immuno-suppressive treatment	autoimmune reaction causing major grade 4 organ dysfunction; progressive and irreversible reaction; long-term adminis-tration of high-dose immunosuppressive therapy required

Also consider Hypothyroidism, Colitis, Hemoglobin, Hemolysis.

Adverse Event	0	1	2	3	4
Serum sickness	none	-	-	present	-

Urticaria is graded in the DERMATOLOGY/SKIN category if it occurs as an isolated symptom. If it occurs with other manifestations of allergic or hypersensitivity reaction, grade as Allergic reaction/hypersensitivity.

Adverse Event	0	1	2	3	4
Vasculitis	none	mild, not requiring treatment	symptomatic, requiring medication	requiring steroids	ischemic changes or requiring amputation
Allergy/Immunology- Other (Specify, _____)	none	mild	moderate	severe	life-threatening or disabling

AUDITORY/HEARING

Conductive hearing loss is graded as Middle ear/hearing in the AUDITORY/HEARING category.

Earache is graded in the PAIN category.

Adverse Event	0	1	2	3	4
External auditory canal	normal	external otitis with erythema or dry desquamation	external otitis with moist desquamation	external otitis with discharge, mastoiditis	necrosis of the canal, soft tissue, or bone

Note: Changes associated with radiation to external ear (pinnae) are graded under Radiation dermatitis in the DERMATOLOGY/SKIN category.

Adverse Event	0	1	2	3	4
Inner ear/hearing	normal	hearing loss on audiometry only	tinnitus or hearing loss, not requiring hearing aid or treatment	tinnitus or hearing loss, correctable with hearing aid or treatment	severe unilateral or bilateral hearing loss (deafness), not correctable
Middle ear/hearing	normal	serous otitis without subjective decrease in hearing	serous otitis or infection requiring medical intervention; subjective decrease in hearing; rupture of tympanic membrane with discharge	otitis with discharge, mastoiditis, or conductive hearing loss	necrosis of the canal, soft tissue, or bone
Auditory/Hearing- Other (Specify, _____)	normal	mild	moderate	severe	life-threatening or disabling

(Continued on next page)

Adverse Event	Grade 0	Grade 1	Grade 2	Grade 3	Grade 4

BLOOD/BONE MARROW

Adverse Event	0	1	2	3	4
Bone marrow cellularity	normal for age	mildly hypocellular or ≤ 25% reduction from normal cellularity for age	moderately hypo-cellular or > 25–≤ 50% reduction from normal cellularity for age or > 2 but < 4 weeks to recovery of normal bone marrow cellularity	severely hypocellular or > 50–≤ 75% reduction in cellularity for age or 4–6 weeks to recovery of normal bone marrow cellularity	aplasia or >6 weeks to recovery of normal bone marrow cellularity

Normal ranges:

children (≤ 18 years)	*90% cellularity average*				
younger adults (19–59)	60–70% cellularity average				
older adults (≥ 60 years)	50% cellularity average				

Note: Grade Bone marrow cellularity only for changes related to treatment not disease.

Adverse Event	0	1	2	3	4
CD4 count	WNL	< LLN–500/mm³	200–< 500/mm³	50–< 200/mm³	< 50/mm³
Haptoglobin	normal	decreased	-	absent	-
Hemoglobin (Hgb)	WNL	< LLN–10.0 g/dl < LLN–100 g/L < LLN–6.2 mmol/L	8.0–< 10.0 g/dl 80–< 100 g/L 4.9–< 6.2 mmol/L	65–< 80 g/L 65–80 g/L 4.0–< 4.9 mmol/L	< 6.5 g/dl < 65 g/L < 4.0 mmol/L
For leukemia studies or bone marrow infiltrative/myeloph-thisic processes, if specified in the protocol.	WNL	10–< 25% decrease from pretreatment	25–< 50% decrease from pretreatment	50–< 75% decrease from pretreatment	≥ 75% decrease from pretreatment
Hemolysis (e.g., immune hemolytic anemia, drug-related hemolysis, other)	none	only laboratory evidence of hemolysis [e.g., direct antiglobu-lin test (DAT, Coombs') schistocytes]	evidence of red cell destruction and ≥ 2g decrease in hemoglo-bin, no transfusion	requiring transfusion and/or medical intervention (e.g., steroids)	catastrophic consequences of hemolysis (e.g., renal failure, hypotension, bronchospasm, emergency splenectomy)

Also consider Haptoglobin, Hemoglobin

Adverse Event	0	1	2	3	4
Leukocytes (total WBC)	WNL	< LLN–3.0 x 10⁹/L < LLN–3,000/mm³	≥ 2.0–< 3.0 x 10⁹/L ≥ 2,000–< 3,000/mm³	≥ 1.0–< 2.0 x 10⁹/L ≥ 1,000–< 2,000/mm³	< 1.0 x 10⁹/L < 1,000/mm³
For BMT studies, if specified in the protocol.	WNL	≥ 2.0–< 3.0 X 10⁹/L ≥ 2,000–< 3,000/mm³	≥ 1.0–< 2.0 x 10⁹/L ≥ 1,000–2,000/mm³	≥ 0.5–< 1.0 x 10⁹/L ≥ 500–< 1,000/mm³	< 0.5 x 10⁹/L < 500/mm³

For pediatric BMT studies (using age, race, and sex normal values), if specified in the protocol.

		≥ 75–< 100% LLN	*≥ 50 - < 75% LLN*	*≥ 25 - 50% LLN*	*< 25% LLN*

Adverse Event	0	1	2	3	4
Lymphopenia	WNL	< LLN–1.0 x 10⁹/L < LLN–1,000/mm³	≥ 0.5–< 1.0 x 10⁹/L ≥ 500–< 1,000/mm³	< 0.5 x 10⁹/L < 500/mm³	-

For pediatric BMT studies (using age, race, and sex normal values), if specified in the protocol.

		≥ 75–< 100%LLN	*≥ 50–< 75%LLN*	*≥ 25–< 50%LLN*	*< 25%LLN*

(Continued on next page)

APPENDICES

Appendix 1. National Cancer Institute Common Toxicity Criteria (CTC) *(Continued)*

Adverse Event	0	Grade 1	Grade 2	Grade 3	Grade 4
Neutrophils/ granulocytes (ANC/AGC)	WNL	$\geq 1.5-< 2.0$ x 10^9/L $\geq 1500-< 2{,}000$/mm³	$\geq 1.0-< 1.5$ x 10^9/L $\geq 1{,}000-< 1{,}500$/mm³	$\geq 0.5-< 1.0$ x 10^9/L $\geq 500-< 1{,}000$/mm³	< 0.5 x 10^9/L < 500/mm³
For BMT studies, if specified in the protocol.	WNL	$\geq 1.0-< 1.5$ x 10^9/L $\geq 1{,}000-< 1{,}500$/mm³	$\geq 0.5-< 1.0$ x 10^9/L $\geq 500-< 1{,}000$/mm³	$\geq 0.1-< 0.5$ x 10^9/L $\geq 100-< 500$/mm³	< 0.1 x 10^9/L < 100/mm³
For leukemia studies or bone marrow infiltrative/myelophthisic process if specified in the protocol.	WNL	$10-< 25\%$ decrease from baseline	$25-< 50\%$ decrease from baseline	$50-< 75\%$ decrease from baseline	$\geq 75\%$ decrease from baseline
Platelets	WNL	$< $ LLN-75.0 x 10^9/L $<$ LLN$-7{,}5000$/mm³	$\geq 50.0-< 75.0$ x 10^9/L $\geq 50{,}000-< 75{,}000$/mm³	$\geq 10.0-< 50.0$ x 10^9/L $\geq 10{,}000-< 50{,}000$/mm³	< 10.0 x 10^9/L $< 10{,}000$/mm³
For BMT studies, if specified in the protocol.	WNL	$\geq 50.0-< 75.0$ x 10^9/L $\geq 50{,}000-< 75{,}000$/mm³	$\geq 20.0-< 50.0$ x 10^9/L $\geq 20{,}000-< 50{,}000$/mm³	$\geq 10.0-< 20.0$ x 10^9/L $\geq 10{,}000-< 20{,}000$/mm³	< 10.0 x 10^9/L $< 10{,}000$/mm³
For leukemia studies or bone marrow infiltrative/myelophthisic process, if specified in the protocol.	WNL	$10-< 25\%$ decrease from baseline	$25-< 50\%$ decrease from baseline	$50-< 75\%$ decrease from baseline	$\geq 75\%$ decrease from baseline
Transfusion: Platelets	none	-	-	yes	platelet transfusions and other measures required to improve platelet increment; platelet transfusion refractoriness associated with life-threatening bleeding (e.g., HLA or cross matched platelet transfusions)
For BMT studies, if specified in the protocol.	none	1 platelet transfusion in 24 hours	2 platelet transfusions in 24 hours	≥ 3 platelet transfusions in 24 hours	platelet transfusions and other measures required to improve platelet increment; platelet transfusion refractoriness associated with life-threatening bleeding (e.g., HLA or cross matched platelet transfusions)
Also consider Platelets.					
Transfusion: pRBCs	none	-	-	Yes	-
For BMT studies, if specified in the protocol.	none	≤ 2 u pRBC ($\leq 15cc/kg$) in 24 hours elective or planned	3 u pRBC ($> 15 \leq 30cc/kg$) in 24 hours elective or planned	≥ 4 u pRBC ($> 30cc/kg$) in 24 hours	hemorrhage or hemolysis associated with life-threatening anemia; medical intervention required to improve hemoglobin
For pediatric BMT studies, if specified in the protocol.	none	$\leq 15mL/kg$ in 24 hours elective or planned	$>15-\leq 30mL/kg$ in 24 hours elective or planned	$> 30mL/kg$ in 24 hours	
Also consider Hemoglobin.					
Blood/bone marrow-other (Specify, _____)	none	mild	moderate	severe	life-threatening or disabling

(Continued on next page)

Appendix 1. National Cancer Institute Common Toxicity Criteria (CTC) *(Continued)*

Adverse Event	Grade 0	1	2	3	4
CARDIOVASCULAR (ARRHYTHMIA)					
Conduction abnormality/ atrioventricular heart block	none	asymptomatic, not requiring treatment (e.g., Mobitz type I second-degree AV block, Wenckebach)	symptomatic, but not requiring treatment	symptomatic and requiring treatment (e.g., Mobitz type II second-degree AV block, third-degree AV block)	life-threatening (e.g., arrhythmia associated with CHF, hypotension, syncope, shock)
Nodal/junctional arrhythmia/ dysrhythmia	none	asymptomatic, not requiring treatment	symptomatic, but not requiring treatment	symptomatic and requiring treatment	life-threatening (e.g., arrhythmia associated with CHF, hypotension, syncope, shock)
Palpitations	none	present	-	-	-
Note: Grade palpitations <u>only</u> in the absence of a documented arrhythmia.					
Prolonged QTc interval (QTc > 0.48 seconds)	none	asymptomatic, not requiring treatment	symptomatic, but not requiring treatment	symptomatic and requiring treatment	life-threatening (e.g., arrhythmia associated with CHF, hypotension, syncope, shock)
Sinus bradycardia	none	asymptomatic, not requiring treatment	symptomatic, but not requiring treatment	symptomatic and requiring treatment	life-threatening (e.g., arrhythmia associated with CHF, hypotension, syncope, shock)
Sinus tachycardia	none	asymptomatic, not requiring treatment	symptomatic, but not requiring treatment	symptomatic and requiring treatment of underlying cause	-
Supraventricular arrhythmias (SVT/ atrial fibrillation/ flutter)	none	asymptomatic, not requiring treatment	symptomatic, but not requiring treatment	symptomatic and requiring treatment	life-threatening (e.g., arrhythmia associated with CHF, hypotension, syncope, shock)
Syncope (fainting) is graded in the NEUROLOGY category.					
Vasovagal episode	none	-	present without loss of consciousness	present with loss of consciousness	-
Ventricular arrhythmia (PVCs/bigeminy/trigeminy/ ventricular tachycardia)	none	asymptomatic, not requiring treatment	symptomatic, but not requiring treatment	symptomatic and requiring treatment	life-threatening (e.g., arrhythmia associated with CHF, hypotension, syncope, shock)
Cardiovascular/ Arrhythmia-Other (Specify, _____)	none	asymptomatic, not requiring treatment	symptomatic, but not requiring treatment	symptomatic, and requiring treatment of underlying cause	life-threatening (e.g., arrhythmia associated with CHF, hypotension, syncope, shock)
CARDIOVASCULAR (GENERAL)					
Acute vascular leak syndrome	absent	-	symptomatic, but not requiring fluid support	respiratory compromise or requiring fluids	life-threatening; requiring pressor support and/or ventilatory support
Cardiac—ischemia/ infarction	none	non-specific T-wave flattening or changes	asymptomatic, ST- and T-wave changes suggesting ischemia	angina without evidence of infarction	acute myocardial infarction

(Continued on next page)

Adverse Event	Grade 0	Grade 1	Grade 2	Grade 3	Grade 4
	0	**1**	**2**	**3**	**4**
Cardiac left ventricular function	normal	asymptomatic decline of resting ejection fraction of $\geq$ 10% but < 20% of baseline value; shortening fraction $\geq$ 24% but < 30%	asymptomatic but resting ejection fraction below LLN for laboratory or decline of resting ejection fraction $\geq$ 20% of baseline value; < 24% shortening fraction	CHF responsive to treatment	severe or refractory CHF or requiring intubation

CNS cerebrovascular ischemia is graded in the NEUROLOGY category.

Adverse Event	0	1	2	3	4
Cardiac troponin I (cTnI)	normal	-	-	levels consistent with unstable angina as defined by the manufacturer	levels consistent with myocardial infarction as defined by the manufacturer
Cardiac troponin T (cTnT)	normal	$\geq$ 0.03–< 0.05 ng/ml	$\geq$ 0.05–< 0.1 ng/ml	$\geq$ 0.1–< 0.2 ng/ml	$\geq$ 0.2 ng/ml
Edema	none	asymptomatic, not requiring therapy	symptomatic, requiring therapy	symptomatic edema limiting function and unresponsive to therapy or requiring drug discontinuation	anasarca (severe generalized edema)
Hypertension	none	asymptomatic, transient increase by > 20 mmHg (diastolic) or to > 150/100* if previously WNL; not requiring treatment	recurrent or persistent or symptomatic increase by > 20 mmHg (diastolic) or to > 150/100* if previously WNL; not requiring treatment	requiring therapy or more intensive therapy than previously	hypertensive crisis

*Note: For pediatric patients, use age-and sex-appropriate normal values > 95th percentile ULN.

Adverse Event	0	1	2	3	4
Hypotension	none	changes, but not requiring therapy (including transient orthostatic hypotension)	requiring brief fluid replacement or other therapy but not hospitalization; no physiologic consequences	requiring therapy and sustained medical attention, but resolves without persisting physiologic consequences	shock (associated with acidemia and impairing vital organ function due to tissue hypoperfusion)

Also consider Syncope (fainting).

Notes: Angina or MI is graded as Cardiac-ischemia/infarction in the CARDIOVASCULAR (GENERAL) category.

For pediatric patients, systolic BP 65 mmHg or less in infants up to 1 year old and 70 mmHg or less in children older than 1 year of age, use two successive or three measurements in 24 hours.

Adverse Event	0	1	2	3	4
Myocarditis	none	-	-	CHF responsive to treatment	severe or refractory CHF
Operative injury of vein/artery	none	primary suture repair for injury, but not requiring transfusion	primary suture repair for injury, requiring transfusion	vascular occlusion requiring surgery or bypass for injury	myocardial infarction; resection of organ (e.g., bowel, limb)
Pericardial effusion/ pericarditis	none	asymptomatic effusion, not requiring treatment	pericarditis (rub, ECG changes, and/or chest pain)	with physiologic consequences	tamponade (drainage or pericardial window required)
Peripheral arterial ischemia	none	-	brief episode of ischemia managed non-surgically and without permanent deficit	requiring surgical intervention	life-threatening or with permanent functional deficit (e.g., amputation)
Phlebitis (superficial)	none	-	present	-	-

Notes: Injection site reaction is graded in the DERMATOLOGY/SKIN category.

Thrombosis/embolism is graded in the CARDIOVASCULAR (GENERAL) category.

Appendix 1. National Cancer Institute Common Toxicity Criteria (CTC) *(Continued)*

(Continued on next page)

Appendix 1. National Cancer Institute Common Toxicity Criteria (CTC) *(Continued)*					
Adverse Event	**0**	**1**	**Grade 2**	**3**	**4**
Syncope (fainting) is graded in the NEUROLOGY category.					
Thrombosis/ embolism	none	-	deep vein thrombosis, not requiring antico-agulant therapy	deep vein thrombosis, requiring anticoagu-lant therapy	embolic event including pulmonary embolism
Vein/artery operative injury is graded as Operative injury of vein/artery in the CARDIOVASCULAR (GENERAL) category.					
Visceral arterial ischemia (non-myocardial)	none	-	brief episode of ischemia managed nonsurgically and without permanent deficit	requiring surgical intervention	life-threatening or with permanent functional deficit (e.g., resection of ileum)
Cardiovascular/ General-Other (Specify, _____)	none	mild	moderate	severe	life-threatening or disabling
COAGULATION					
Note: See the HEMORRHAGE category for grading the severity of bleeding events.					
DIC (dissem-inated intravascular coagulation)	absent	-	-	laboratory findings present with <u>no</u> bleeding	laboratory findings <u>and</u> bleeding
Also consider Platelets. Note: Must have increased fibrin split products or D-dimer in order to grade as DIC.					
Fibrinogen	WNL	≥ 0.75–< 1.0 x LLN	≥ 0.5– < 0.75 x LLN	≥ 0.25–< 0.5 x LLN	< 0.25 x LLN
For leukemia studies or bone marrow infiltrative/myeloph-thisic process, if specified in the protocol.	WNL	< 20% decrease from pretreatment value or LLN	≥ 20–< 40% decrease from pretreatment value or LLN	≥ 40–< 70% decrease from pretreatment value or LLN	< 50 mg
Partial thromboplas-tin time (PTT)	WNL	> ULN–≤ 1.5 x ULN	> 1.5–≤ 2 x ULN	> 2 x ULN	-
Phlebitis is graded in the CARDIOVASCULAR (GENERAL) category.					
Prothrombin time (PT)	WNL	> ULN–≤ 1.5 x ULN	> 1.5–≤ 2 x ULN	> 2 x ULN	-
Thrombosis/embolism is graded in the CARDIOVASCULAR (GENERAL) category.					
Thrombotic microangiopathy (e.g., thrombotic thrombocytopenic purpura/TTP or hemolytic uremic syndrome/HUS)	absent	-	-	laboratory findings present without clinical consequences	laboratory findings and clinical conse-quences, (e.g., CNS hemorrhage/bleed-ing or thrombosis/ embolism or renal failure) requiring ther-apeutic intervention
For BMT studies, if specified in the protocol.	-	evidence of RBC destruction (schistocy-tosis) without clinical consequences	evidence of RBC destruction with elevated creatinine (≤ 3 x ULN)	evidence of RBC destruction with creatinine (> 3 x ULN) not requiring dialysis	evidence of RBC destruction with renal failure requiring dialysis and/or encephalopathy
Also consider Hemoglobin (Hgb), Platelets, Creatinine. Note: Must have microangiopathic changes on blood smear (e.g., schistocytes, helmet cells, red cell fragments).					
Coagulation-Other (Specify, _____)	none	mild	moderate	severe	life-threatening or disabling

(Continued on next page)

APPENDICES

Adverse Event	Grade 0	1	2	3	4

CONSTITUTIONAL SYMPTOMS

Adverse Event	0	1	2	3	4
Fatigue (lethargy, malaise, asthenia)	none	increased fatigue over baseline, but not altering normal activities	moderate (e.g., decrease in performance status by 1 ECOG level or 20% Karnofsky or *Lansky*) or causing difficulty performing some activities	severe (e.g., decrease in performance status by ≥ 2 ECOG levels or 40% Karnofsky or *Lansky*) or loss of ability to perform some activities	bedridden or disabling
Fever (in the absence of neutropenia, where neutropenia is defined as AGC < 1.0 x 10⁹/L)	none	38.0–39.0°C (100.4–102.2°F)	39.1–40.0°C (102.3–104.0°F)	> 40.0°C (> 104.0°F) for < 24hrs	> 40.0°C (> 104.0°F) for > 24hrs

Also consider Allergic reaction/hypersensitivity.

Note: The temperature measurements listed above are oral or tympanic.

Hot flashes/flushes are graded in the ENDOCRINE category.

Adverse Event	0	1	2	3	4
Rigors, chills	none	mild, requiring symptomatic treatment (e.g., blanket) or non-narcotic medication	severe and/or prolonged, requiring narcotic medication	not responsive to narcotic medication	-
Sweating (diaphoresis)	none	mild and occasional	frequent or drenching	-	-
Weight gain	< 5%	5–< 10%	10–< 20%	≥ 20%	-

Also consider Ascites, Edema, Pleural effusion (non-malignant).

Adverse Event	0	1	2	3	4
Weight gain associated with Veno-Occlusive Disease (VOD), for BMT studies, if specified in the protocol.	< 2%	≥ 2–< 5%	≥ 5–< 10%	≥ 10% or as ascites	≥ 10% or fluid retention resulting in pulmonary failure

Also consider Ascites, Edema Pleural effusion (non-malignant).

Adverse Event	0	1	2	3	4
Weight loss	< 5%	5–< 10%	10–< 20%	≥ 20%	-

Also consider Vomiting, Dehydration, Diarrhea.

Adverse Event	0	1	2	3	4
Constitutional Symptoms-Other (Specify, _____)	none	mild	moderate	severe	life-threatening or disabling

DERMATOLOGY/SKIN

Adverse Event	0	1	2	3	4
Alopecia	normal	mild hair loss	pronounced hair loss	-	-
Bruising (in absence of grade 3 or 4 thrombocytopenia)	none	localized or in dependent area	generalized	-	-

Note: Bruising resulting from grade 3 or 4 thrombocytopenia is graded as Petechiae/purpura and Hemorrhage/bleeding with grade 3 or 4 thrombocytopenia in the HEMORRHAGE category, not in the DERMATOLOGY/SKIN category.

Adverse Event	0	1	2	3	4
Dry skin	normal	controlled with emollients	not controlled with emollients	-	-
Erythema multiforme (e.g., Stevens-Johnson syndrome, toxic epidermal necrolysis)	absent	-	scattered, but not generalized eruption	severe or requiring IV fluids (e.g., generalized rash or painful stomatitis)	life-threatening (e.g., exfoliative or ulcerating dermatitis or requiring enteral or parenteral nutritional support)

(Continued on next page)

APPENDICES

Appendix 1. National Cancer Institute Common Toxicity Criteria (CTC) *(Continued)*

Adverse Event	0	1	2	3	4
			Grade		
Flushing	absent	present	-	-	-
Hand-foot skin reaction	none	skin changes or dermatitis without pain (e.g., erythema, peeling)	skin changes with pain, not interfering with function	skin changes with pain, interfering with function	-
Injection site reaction	none	pain or itching or erythema	pain or swelling, with inflammation or phlebitis	ulceration or necrosis that is severe or prolonged, or requiring surgery	-
Nail changes	normal	discoloration or ridging (koilonychia) or pitting partial or complete	loss of nail(s) or pain in nailbeds	-	-

Petechiae is graded in the HEMORRHAGE category.

Adverse Event	0	1	2	3	4
Photosensitivity	none	painless erythema	painful erythema	erythema with desquamation	-
Pigmentation changes (e.g., vitiligo)	none	localized pigmentation changes	generalized pigmentation changes	-	-
Pruritus	none	mild or localized, relieved spontaneously or by local measures	intense or widespread, relieved spontaneously or by systemic measures	intense or widespread and poorly controlled despite treatment	-

Purpura is graded in the HEMORRHAGE category.

Adverse Event	0	1	2	3	4
Radiation dermatitis	none	faint erythema or dry desquamation	moderate to brisk erythema or a patchy moist desquamation, mostly confined to skin folds and creases; moderate edema	confluent moist desquamation, ≥ 1.5 cm diameter, not confined to skin folds; pitting edema	skin necrosis or ulceration of full thickness dermis; may include bleeding not induced by minor trauma or abrasion

Note: Pain associated with radiation dermatitis is graded separately in the PAIN category as Pain due to radiation.

Adverse Event	0	1	2	3	4
Radiation recall reaction (reaction following chemotherapy in the absence of additional radiation therapy that occurs in a previous radiation port)	none	faint erythema or dry desquamation	moderate to brisk erythema or a patchy moist desquamation, mostly confined to skin folds and creases; moderate edema	confluent moist desquamation, ≥ 1.5 cm diameter, not confined to skin folds; pitting edema	skin necrosis or ulceration of full thickness dermis; may include bleeding not induced by minor trauma or abrasion
Rash/desquamation	none	macular or papular eruption or erythema without associated symptoms	macular or papular eruption or erythema with pruritus or other associated symptoms covering < 50% of body surface or localized desquamation or other lesions covering < 50% of body surface area	symptomatic generalized erythroderma or macular, papular, or vesicular eruption or desquamation covering ≥ 50% of body surface area	generalized exfoliative dermatitis or ulcerative dermatitis

Also consider Allergic reaction/hypersensitivity.
Note: Stevens-Johnson syndrome is graded separatley as Erythema multiforme in DERMATOLOGY/SKIN category.

Adverse Event	0	1	2	3	4
Rash/Dermatitis, focal (associated with high-dose chemotherapy and bone marrow transplant)	none	faint erythema or dry desquamation	moderate to brisk erythema or a patchy moist desquamation, mostly confined to skin folds and creases; moderate edema	confluent moist desquamation, ≥ 1.5 cm diameter, not confined to skin folds; pitting edema	skin necrosis or ulceration of full thickness dermis; may include spontaneous bleeding not induced by minor trauma or abrasion

(Continued on next page)

Appendix 1. National Cancer Institute Common Toxicity Criteria (CTC) *(Continued)*

Adverse Event	Grade 0	1	2	3	4
Rash/dermatitis associated with high dose chemotherapy or BMT studies. Rash/desquamation associated with graft versus host disease (GVHD) for BMT studies is specified in the protocol.	none	macular or papular eruption or erythema covering < 25% of body surface area without associated symptoms	macular or papular eruption or erythema with pruritus or other associated symptoms covering ≥ 25–< 50% of body surface or localized desquamation or other lesions covering ≥ 25–< 50% of body surface area	symptomatic generalized erythroderma or symptomatic macular, papular, or vesicular eruption, with bullous formation, or desquamation covering ≥ 50% of body surface area	generalized exfoliative dermatitis or ulcerative dermatitis or bullous formation

Also consider Allergic reaction/hypersensitivity.

Note: Stevens-Johnson syndrome is graded separately as Erythema multiforme in the DERMATOLOGY/SKIN category.

Adverse Event	0	1	2	3	4
Urticaria (hives, welts, wheals)	none	requiring no medication	requiring PO or topical treatment or IV medication or steroids for < 24 hours	requiring IV medication or steroids for ≥24 hours	-
Wound-infectious	none	cellulitis	superficial infection	infection requiring IV antibiotics	necrotizing fasciitis
Wound-non-infectious	none	incisional separation	incisional hernia	fascial disruption without evisceration	fascial disruption with evisceration
Dermatology/Skin-Other (Specify, _____)	none	mild	moderate	severe	life-threatening or disabling

ENDOCRINE

Adverse Event	0	1	2	3	4
Cushingoid appearance (e.g., moon face, buffalo hump, centripetal obesity, cutaneous striae)	absent	-	present	-	-

Also consider Hyperglycemia, Hypokalemia.

Adverse Event	0	1	2	3	4
Feminization of male	absent	-	-	present	-
Gynecomastia	none	mild	pronounced or painful	pronounced or painful and requiring surgery	-
Hot flashes/flushes	none	mild or no more than 1 per day	moderate and greater than 1 per day	-	-
Hypothyroidism	absent	asymptomatic, TSH elevated, no therapy given	symptomatic or thyroid replacement treatment given	patient hospitalized for manifestations of hypothyroidism	myxedema coma
Masculinization of female	absent	-	-	present	-
SIADH (syndrome of inappropriate anti-diuretic hormone)	absent	-	-	present	-
Endocrine-Other (Specify, _____)	none	mild	moderate	severe	life-threatening or disabling

GASTROINTESTINAL

Amylase is graded in the METABOLIC/LABORATORY category.

Adverse Event	0	1	2	3	4
Anorexia	none	loss of appetite	oral intake significantly decreased	requiring IV fluids	requiring feeding tube or parenteral nutrition

(Continued on next page)

Appendix 1. National Cancer Institute Common Toxicity Criteria (CTC) *(Continued)*

Adverse Event	0	1	2	3	4
Ascites (non-malignant)	none	asymptomatic	symptomatic, requiring diuretics	symptomatic, requiring therapeutic paracentesis	life-threatening physiologic consequences
Colitis	none	-	abdominal pain with mucus and/or blood in stool	abdominal pain, fever, change in bowel habits with ileus or peritoneal signs, and radiographic or biopsy documentation	perforation or requiring surgery or toxic megacolon

Also consider Hemorrhage/bleeding with grade 3 or 4 thrombocytopenia, Hemorrhage/bleeding without grade 3 or 4 thrombocytopenia, Melena/GI bleeding, Rectal bleeding/hematochezia, Hypotension.

Adverse Event	0	1	2	3	4
Constipation	none	requiring stool softener or dietary modification	requiring laxatives	obstipation requiring manual evacuation or enema	obstruction or toxic megacolon
Dehydration	none	dry mucous membranes and/or diminished skin turgor	requiring IV fluid replacement (brief)	requiring IV fluid replacement (sustained)	physiologic consequences requiring intensive care; hemodynamic collapse

Also consider Diarrhea, Vomiting, Stomatitis/pharyngitis (oral/pharyngeal mucositis) Hypotension.

Adverse Event	0	1	2	3	4
Diarrhea Patients without colostomy:	none	increase of < 4 stools/ day over pre-treatment	increase of 4–6 stools/ day, or nocturnal stools	increase of ≥ 7 stools/ day or incontinence; or need for parenteral support for dehydration	physiologic consequences requiring intensive care; or hemodynamic collapse
Patients with colostomy:	none	mild increase in loose, watery colostomy output compared with pretreatment	moderate increase in loose, watery colostomy output compared with pretreatment, but not interfering with normal activity	severe increase in loose, watery colostomy output compared with pretreatment, interfering with normal activity	physiologic consequences, requiring intensive care; or hemodynamic collapse
For BMT diarrhea associated with GVHD studies, if specified in the protocol.	none	> 500–≤ 1,000 ml of diarrhea/day	> 1,000–≤ 1,500 ml of diarrhea/day	> 1,500 ml of diarrhea/ day	severe abdominal pain with or without ileus
For Pediatric BMT studies, if specified in the protocol.		*> 5–≤ 10 ml/kg of diarrhea/day*	*> 10–≤ 15 ml/kg of diarrhea/day*	*> 15 ml/kg of diarrhea/ day*	*-*

Also consider Hemorrhage/bleeding with grade 3 or 4 thrombocytopenia, Hemorrhage/bleeding without grade 3 or 4 thrombocytopenia, Pain, Dehydration, Hypotension.

Adverse Event	0	1	2	3	4
Duodenal ulcer (requires radiographic or endoscopic documentation)	none	-	requiring medical management or non-surgical treatment	uncontrolled by outpatient medical management; requiring hospitalization	perforation or bleeding, requiring emergency surgery
Dyspepsia/ heartburn	none	mild	moderate	severe	-
Dysphagia, esophagitis, odynophagia (painful swallowing)	none	mild dysphagia, but can eat regular diet	dysphagia, requiring predominantly pureed, soft, or liquid diet	dysphagia, requiring IV hydration	complete obstruction (cannot swallow saliva) requiring enteral or parenteral nutritional support, or perforation

Note: If the adverse event is radiation-related, grade <u>either</u> under Dysphagia—esophageal related to radiation <u>or</u> Dysphagia—pharyngeal related to radiation.

(Continued on next page)

APPENDICES

Adverse Event	0	1	2	3	4
			Grade		
Dysphagia— esophageal related to radiation	none	mild dysphagia, but can eat regular diet	dysphagia, requiring predominantly liquid, pureed, or soft diet	dysphagia requiring feeding tube, IV hydration, or hyper-alimentation	complete obstruc-tion (cannot swallow saliva); ulceration with bleeding not induced by minor trauma or abrasion or perforation
Also consider Pain due to radiation, Mucositis due to radiation. Note: Fistula is graded separately as Fistula—esophageal.					
Dysphagia— pharyngeal related to radiation	none	mild dysphagia, but can eat regular diet	dysphagia, requiring predominantly pureed, soft, or liquid diet	dysphagia, requiring feeding tube, IV hydration or hyper-alimentation	complete obstruc-tion (cannot swallow saliva); ulceration with bleeding not induced by minor trauma or abrasion or perforation
Also consider Pain due to radiation, Mucositis due to radiation. Note: Fistula is graded separately as Fistula—pharyngeal.					
Fistula—esophageal	none	-	-	present	requiring surgery
Fistula—intestinal	none	-	-	present	requiring surgery
Fistula—pharyngeal	none	-	-	present	requiring surgery
Fistula—rectal/anal	none	-	-	present	requiring surgery
Flatulence	none	mild	moderate	-	-
Gastric ulcer (requires radio-graphic or endo-scopic documenta-tion)	none	-	requiring medical management or non-surgical treatment	bleeding without perforation, uncon-trolled by outpatient medical management, requiring hospitaliza-tion or surgery	perforation or bleeding, requiring emergency surgery
Also consider Hemorrhage/bleeding with grade 3 or 4 thrombocytopenia, Hemorrhage/bleeding without grade 3 or 4 thrombocytopenia.					
Gastritis	none	-	requiring medical management or non-surgical treatment	uncontrolled by out-patient medical management, requiring hospitaliza-tion or surgery	life-threatening bleeding, requiring emergency surgery
Also consider Hemorrhage/bleeding with grade 3 or 4 thrombocytopenia, Hemorrhage/bleeding without grade 3 or 4 thrombocytopenia.					
Hematemesis is graded in the HEMORRHAGE category.					
Hematochezia is graded in the HEMORRHAGE category as Rectal bleeding/hematochezia.					
Ileus (or neuro-constipation)	none	-	intermittent, not requiring intervention	requiring non-surgical intervention	requiring surgery
Mouth dryness	normal	mild	moderate	-	-

Mucositis

Note: Mucositis not due to radiation is graded in the GASTROINTESTINAL category for specific sites: Colitis, Esophagitis, Gastritis, Stomati-tis/pharyngitis (oral/pharyngeal mucositis), and Typhlitis; or the RENAL/GENITOURINARY category for Vaginitis.

Radiation-related mucositis is graded as Mucositis due to radiation.

(Continued on next page)

APPENDICES

Adverse Event	0	1	2	3	4
			Grade		
Mucositis due to radiation	none	erythema of the mucosa	patchy pseudomembranous reaction (patches generally ≤ 1.5 cm in diameter and non-contiguous)	confluent pseudomembranous reaction (contiguous patches generally > 1.5 cm in diameter)	necrosis or deep ulceration; may include bleeding not induced by minor trauma or abrasion

Also consider Pain due to radiation.

Notes: Grade radiation mucositis of the larynx here.

Dysphagia related to radiation is also graded as <u>either</u> Dysphagia—esophageal related to radiation <u>or</u> Dysphagia—pharyngeal related to radiation, depending on the site of treatment.

Nausea	none	able to eat	oral intake significantly decreased	no significant intake, requiring IV fluids	-
Pancreatitis	none	-	-	abdominal pain with pancreatic enzyme elevation	complicated by shock (acute circulatory failure)

Also consider Hypotension.

Note: Amylase is graded in the METABOLIC/LABORATORY category.

Pharyngitis is graded in the GASTROINTESTINAL category as Stomatitis/pharyngitis (oral/pharyngeal mucositis).

Proctitis	none	increased stool frequency, occasional blood-streaked stools, or rectal discomfort (including hemorrhoids), not requiring medication	increased stool frequency, bleeding, mucus discharge, or rectal discomfort requiring medication; anal fissure	increased stool frequency/diarrhea, requiring parenteral support; rectal bleeding, requiring transfusion; or persistent mucus discharge, necessitating pads	perforation, bleeding or necrosis or other life-threatening complication requiring surgical intervention (e.g., colostomy)

Also consider Hemorrhage/bleeding with grade 3 or 4 thrombocytopenia, Hemorrhage/bleeding without grade 3 or 4 thrombocytopenia, Pain due to radiation.

Notes: Fistula is graded separately as Fistula—rectal/anal.

Proctitis occurring more than 90 days after the start of radiation therapy is graded in the RTOG/EORTC Late Radiation Morbidity Scoring Scheme.

Salivary gland changes	none	slightly thickened saliva/may have slightly altered taste (e.g., metallic); additional fluids may be required	thick, ropy, sticky saliva; markedly altered taste; alteration in diet required	-	acute salivary gland necrosis
Sense of smell	normal	slightly altered	markedly altered	-	-
Stomatitis/pharyngitis (oral/pharyngeal mucositis)	none	painless ulcers, erythema, or mild soreness in the absence of lesions	painful erythema, edema, or ulcers but can eat or swallow	painful erythema, edema, or ulcers requiring IV hydration	severe ulceration or requires parenteral or enteral nutritional support or prophylactic intubation
For BMT studies, if specified in the protocol.	none	painless ulcers, erythema, or mild soreness in the absence of lesions	painful erythema, edema, or ulcers but can swallow	painful erythema, edema, or ulcers preventing swallowing or requiring hydration or parenteral (or enteral) nutritional support	severe ulceration requiring prophylactic intubation or resulting in documented aspiration pneumonia

Note: Radiation-related mucositis is graded as Mucositis due to radiation.

Taste disturbance (dysgeusia)	normal	slightly altered	markedly altered	-	-

(Continued on next page)

APPENDICES

Adverse Event	Grade 0	1	2	3	4
Typhlitis (inflammation of the cecum)	none	-	-	abdominal pain, diarrhea, fever, and radiographic or biopsy documentation	perforation, bleeding or necrosis or other life-threatening complication requiring surgical intervention (e.g., colostomy)

Also consider Hemorrhage/bleeding with grade 3 or 4 thrombocytopenia, Hemorrhage/bleeding without grade 3 or 4 thrombocytopenia, Hypotension, Febrile neutropenia.

| Vomiting | none | 1 episode in 24 hours over pretreatment | 2–5 episodes in 24 hours over pretreatment | ≥ 6 episodes in 24 hours over pretreatment; or need for IV fluids | Requiring parenteral nutrition; or physiologic consequences requiring intensive care; hemodynamic collapse |

Also consider Dehydration.

Weight gain is graded in the CONSTITUTIONAL SYMPTOMS category.

Weight loss is graded in the CONSTITUTIONAL SYMPTOMS category.

| Gastrointestinal-Other (Specify, _____) | none | mild | moderate | severe | life-threatening or disabling |

HEMORRHAGE

Notes: Transfusion in this section refers to pRBC infusion.

For <u>any</u> bleeding with grade 3 or 4 platelets (< 50,000), <u>always</u> grade Hemorrhage/bleeding with grade 3 or 4 thrombocytopenia. Also consider platelets, transfusion-pRBC, and transfusion-platelets in addition by grading the site or type of bleeding.

If the site or type of hemorrhage/bleeding is listed, also use the grading that incorporates the site of bleeding: CNS hemorrhage/bleeding, Hematuria, Hematemesis, Hemoptysis, Hemorrhage/bleeding with surgery, Melena/lower GI bleeding, Petechiae/purpura (Hemorrhage/bleeding into skin), Rectal bleeding/hematochezia, Vaginal bleeding.

If the platelet count is ≥ 50,000 and the site or type of bleeding is listed, grade the specific site. If the site or type is <u>not</u> listed and the platelet count is ≥ 50,000, grade Hemorrhage/bleeding without grade 3 or 4 thrombocytopenia and specify the site or type in the OTHER category.

| Hemorrhage/bleeding with grade 3 or 4 thrombocytopenia | none | mild without transfusion | - | requiring transfusion | catastrophic bleeding, requiring major non-elective intervention |

Also consider Platelets, Hemoglobin, Transfusion-platelet, Transfusion-pRBCs or type of bleeding. If the site is not listed, grade as Hemorrhage-Other (Specify site, _____)

Note: This adverse event must be graded for any bleeding with grade 3 or 4 thrombocytopenia.

| Hemorrhage/bleeding without grade 3 or 4 thrombocytopenia | none | mild without transfusion | - | requiring transfusion | catastrophic bleeding requiring major non-elective intervention |

Also consider Platelets, Hemoglobin, Transfusion-platelet, Transfusion-pRBCs. Hemorrhage-Other (Specify site, _____)

Note: Bleeding in the absence of grade 3 or 4 thrombocytopenia is graded here only if the specific site or type of bleeding is not listed elsewhere in the HEMORRHAGE category.

| CNS hemorrhage/bleeding | none | - | - | bleeding noted on CT or other scan with no clinical consequences | hemorrhagic stroke or hemorrhagic vascular event (CVA) with neurologic signs and symptoms |
| Epistaxis | none | mild without transfusion | - | requiring transfusion | catastrophic bleeding, requiring major non-elective intervention |

(Continued on next page)

Adverse Event	0	Grade 1	2	3	4
Hematemesis	none	mild without transfusion	-	requiring transfusion	catastrophic bleeding, requiring major non-elective intervention
Hematuria (in the absence of vaginal bleeding)	none	microscopic only	intermittent gross bleeding, no clots	persistent gross bleeding or clots; may require catheterization or instrumentation, or transfusion	open surgery or necrosis or deep bladder ulceration
Hemoptysis	none	mild without transfusion	-	requiring transfusion	catastrophic bleeding, requiring major non-elective intervention
Hemorrhage/ bleeding associated with surgery	none	mild without transfusion	-	requiring transfusion	catastrophic bleeding, requiring major non-elective intervention
Note: Expected blood loss at the time of surgery is not graded as an adverse event.					
Melena/GI bleeding	none	mild without transfusion	-	requiring transfusion	catastrophic bleeding, requiring major non-elective intervention
Petechiae/purpura (hemorrhage/ bleeding into skin or mucosa)	none	rare petechiae of skin	petechiae or purpura in dependent areas of skin	generalized petechiae or purpura of skin or petechiae of any mucosal site	-
Rectal bleeding/ hematochezia	none	mild without transfusion or medication	persistent, requiring medication (e.g., steroid suppositories) and/or break from radiation treatment	requiring transfusion	catastrophic bleeding, requiring major non-elective intervention
Vaginal bleeding	none	spotting, requiring < 2 pads per day	requiring ≥ 2 pads per day, but not requiring transfusion	requiring transfusion	catastrophic bleeding, requiring major non-elective intervention
Hemorrhage-Other (Specify site, _____)	none	mild without transfusion	-	requiring transfusion	catastrophic bleeding, requiring major non-elective intervention
HEPATIC					
Alkaline phosphatase	WNL	> ULN–2.5 x ULN	> 2.5–5.0 x ULN	> 5.0–20.0 x ULN	> 20.0 x ULN
Bilirubin	WNL	> ULN–1.5 x ULN	> 1.5–3.0 x ULN	> 3.0–10.0 x ULN	> 10.0 x ULN
Bilirubin associated with graft versus host disease (GVHD) for BMT studies, if specified in the protocol. Note: The following criteria are used only for bilirubin associated with graft versus host disease.	normal	≥ 2–< 3 mg/100 ml	≥ 3–< 6 mg/100 ml	≥ 6–< 15 mg/100 ml	≥ 15 mg/100 ml
GGT (g-Glutamyl transpeptidase)	WNL	> ULN–2.5 x ULN	> 2.5–5.0 x ULN	> 5.0–20.0 x ULN	> 20.0 x ULN
Hepatic enlargement	absent	-	-	present	-
Note: Grade Hepatic enlargement only for changes related to adverse events including VOD.					
Hypoalbuminemia	WNL	< LLN–3 g/dl	≥ 2–< 3 g/dl	< 2 g/dl	-

(Continued on next page)

APPENDICES

Appendix 1. National Cancer Institute Common Toxicity Criteria (CTC) *(Continued)*					
Adverse Event	**0**	**1**	**Grade 2**	**3**	**4**
Liver dysfunction/ failure (clinical)	normal	-	-	asterixis	encephalopathy or coma
Portal vein flow	normal	-	decreased portal vein flow	reversal/retrograde portal vein flow	-
SGOT (AST) (serum glutamic oxaloacetic transaminase)	WNL	> ULN–2.5 x ULN	> 2.5–5.0 x ULN	> 5.0–20.0 x ULN	> 20.0 x ULN
SGPT (ALT) (serum glutamic pyruvic transaminase)	WNL	> ULN–2.5 x ULN	> 2.5–5.0 x ULN	> 5.0–20.0 x ULN	> 20.0 x ULN
Hepatic-Other (Specify, _____)	none	mild	moderate	severe	life-threatening or disabling
INFECTION/FEBRILE NEUTROPENIA					
Catheter-related infection	none	mild, no active treatment	moderate, localized infection, requiring local or oral treatment	severe, systemic infection, requiring IV antibiotic or antifungal treatment or hospitalization	life-threatening sepsis (e.g., septic shock)
Febrile neutropenia (fever of unknown origin without clinically or microbiologically documented infection) (ANC < 1.0 x 10^9/L, fever ≥ 38.5°C)	none	-	-	present	life-threatening sepsis (e.g., septic shock)
Also consider Neutrophils. Note: Hypothermia instead of fever may be associated with neutropenia and is graded here.					
Infection (documented clinically or microbiologically) with grade 3 or 4 neutropenia (ANC < 1.0 x 10^9/L)	none	-	-	present	life-threatening sepsis (e.g., septic shock)
Also consider infection. Note: Hypothermia instead of fever may be associated with neutropenia and is graded here. In the absence of documented infection with grade 3 or 4 neutropenia, with fever is graded as Febrile neutropenia.					
Infection with unknown ANC	none	-	-	present	life-threatening sepsis (e.g., septic shock)
Note: This adverse event criterion is used in the rare case when ANC is unknown.					
Infection without neutropenia	none	mild, no active treatment	moderate, localized infection, requiring local or oral treatment	severe, systemic infection, requiring IV antibiotic or antifungal treatment, or hospitalization	life-threatening sepsis (e.g., septic shock)
Also consider Neutrophils.					
Wound-infectious is graded in the DERMATOLOGY/SKIN category.					
Infection/Febrile Neutropenia-Other (Specify, _____)	none	mild	moderate	severe	life-threatening or disabling

(Continued on next page)

Appendix 1. National Cancer Institute Common Toxicity Criteria (CTC) *(Continued)*

Adverse Event	0	Grade 1	2	3	4
LYMPHATICS					
Lymphatics	normal	mild lymphedema	moderate lymphedema requiring compression; lymphocyst	severe lymphedema limiting function; lymphocyst requiring surgery	severe lymphedema limiting function with ulceration
Lymphatics-Other (Specify, _____)	none	mild	moderate	severe	life-threatening or disabling
METABOLIC/LABORATORY					
Acidosis (metabolic or respiratory)	normal	pH < normal, but ≥ 7.3	-	pH < 7.3	pH < 7.3 with life-threatening physiologic consequences
Alkalosis (metabolic or respiratory)	normal	pH > normal, but ≤ 7.5	-	pH > 7.5	pH > 7.5 with life-threatening physiologic consequences
Amylase	WNL	> ULN–1.5 x ULN	> 1.5–2.0 x ULN	> 2.0–5.0 x ULN	> 5.0 x ULN
Bicarbonate	WNL	< LLN–16 mEq/dl	11–15 mEq/dl	8–10 mEq/dl	< 8 mEq/dl
CPK (creatine phosphokinase)	WNL	> ULN–2.5 x ULN	> 2.5–5 x ULN	> 5–10 x ULN	> 10 x ULN
Hypercalcemia	WNL	> ULN–11.5 mg/dl > ULN–2.9 mmol/L	> 11.5–12.5 mg/dl > 2.9–3.1 mmol/L	> 12.5–13.5 mg/dl > 3.1–3.4 mmol/L	> 13.5 mg/dl > 3.4 mmol/L
Hypercholesterolemia	WNL	> ULN–300 mg/dl > ULN–7.75 mmol/L	> 300–400 mg/dl > 7.75–10.34 mmol/L	> 400–500 mg/dl > 10.34–12.92 mmol/L	> 500 mg/dl > 12.92 mmol/L
Hyperglycemia	WNL	> ULN–160 mg/dl > ULN–8.9 mmol/L	> 160–250 mg/dl > 8.9–13.9 mmol/L	> 250–500 mg/dl > 13.9–27.8 mmol/L	> 500 mg/dl > 27.8 mmol/L or acidosis
Hyperkalemia	WNL	> ULN–5.5 mmol/L	> 5.5–6.0 mmol/L	> 6.0–7.0 mmol/L	> 7.0 mmol/L
Hypermagnesemia	WNL	> ULN–3.0 mg/dl > ULN–1.23 mmol/L	-	> 3.0–8.0 mg/dl > 1.23–3.30 mmol/L	> 8.0 mg/dl > 3.30 mmol/L
Hypernatremia	WNL	> ULN–150 mmol/L	> 150–155 mmol/L	> 155–160 mmol/L	> 160 mmol/L
Hypertriglyceridemia	WNL	> ULN–2.5 x ULN	> 2.5–5.0 x ULN	> 5.0–10 x ULN	> 10 x ULN
Hyperuricemia	WNL	> ULN–≤ 10 mg/dl ≤ 0.59 mmol/L without physiologic consequences	-	> ULN–≤ 10 mg/dl ≤ 0.59 mmol/L with physiologic consequences	> 10 mg/dl > 0.59 mmol/L
Also consider Tumor lysis syndrome, Renal failure, Creatinine, Hyperkalemia.					
Hypocalcemia	WNL	< LLN–8.0 mg/dl < LLN–2.0 mmol/L	7.0–< 8.0 mg/dl 1.75–< 2.0 mmol/L	6.0–< 7.0 mg/dl 1.5–< 1.75 mmol/L	< 6.0 mg/dl < 1.5 mmol/L
Hypoglycemia	WNL	< LLN–55 mg/dl < LLN–3.0 mmol/L	40–< 55 mg/dl 2.2–< 3.0 mmol/L	30–< 40 mg/dl 1.7–< 2.2 mmol/L	< 30 mg/dl < 1.7 mmol/L
Hypokalemia	WNL	< LLN–3.0 mmol/L	-	2.5–< 3.0 mmol/L	< 2.5 mmol/L
Hypomagnesemia	WNL	< LLN–1.2 mg/dl < LLN–0.5 mmol/L	0.9–< 1.2 mg/dl 0.4–< 0.5 mmol/L	0.7–< 0.9 mg/dl 0.3–< 0.4 mmol/L	< 0.7 mg/dl < 0.3 mmol/L
Hyponatremia	WNL	< LLN–130 mmol/L	-	120–< 130 mmol/L	< 120 mmol/L
Hypophosphatemia	WNL	< LLN–2.5 mg/dl < LLN–0.8 mmol/L	≥ 2.0–< 2.5 mg/dl ≥ 0.6–< 0.8 mmol/L	≥ 1.0–< 2.0 mg/dl ≥ 0.3–< 0.6 mmol/L	< 1.0 mg/dl < 0.3 mmol/L

(Continued on next page)

Appendix 1. National Cancer Institute Common Toxicity Criteria (CTC) *(Continued)*

Adverse Event	0	1	2	3	4
			Grade		

Hypothyroidism is graded in the ENDOCRINE category.

Adverse Event	0	1	2	3	4
Lipase	WNL	> ULN–1.5 x ULN	> 1.5–2.0 x ULN	> 2.0–5.0 x ULN	> 5.0 x ULN
Metabolic/Laboratory-Other (Specify, _____)	none	mild	moderate	severe	life-threatening or disabling

MUSCULOSKELETAL

Arthralgia is graded in the PAIN category.

Adverse Event	0	1	2	3	4
Arthritis	none	mild pain with inflammation, erythema or joint swelling but not interfering with function	moderate pain with inflammation, erythema, or joint swelling interfering with function, but not interfering with activities of daily living	severe pain with inflammation, erythema, or joint swelling and interfering with activities of daily living	disabling
Muscle weakness (not due to neuropathy)	normal	asymptomatic with weakness on physical exam	symptomatic and interfering with function, but not interfering with activities of daily living	symptomatic and interfering with activities of daily living	bedridden or disabling

Myalgia (tenderness or pain in muscles) is graded in the PAIN category.

Adverse Event	0	1	2	3	4
Myositis (inflammation/damage of muscle)	none	mild pain, not interfering with function	pain interfering with function, but not interfering with activities of daily living	pain interfering with function and interfering with activities of daily living	bedridden or disabling

Also consider CPK.

Note: Myositis implies muscle damage (i.e., elevated CPK).

Adverse Event	0	1	2	3	4
Osteonecrosis (avascular necrosis)	none	asymptomatic and detected by imaging only	symptomatic and interfering with function, but not interfering with	activities of daily living symptomatic and interfering with	activities of daily living symptomatic; or disabling
Musculoskeletal-Other (Specify, _____)	none	mild	moderate	severe	life-threatening or disabling

NEUROLOGY

Aphasia, receptive and/or expressive, is graded under Speech impairment in the NEUROLOGY category.

Adverse Event	0	1	2	3	4
Arachnoiditis/ meningismus/ radiculitis	absent	mild pain not interfering with function	moderate pain interfering with function but not interfering with activities of daily living	severe pain interfering with activities of daily living	unable to function or perform activities of daily living; bedridden; paraplegia

Also consider Headache, Vomiting, Fever.

Adverse Event	0	1	2	3	4
Ataxia (incoordination)	normal	asymptomatic but abnormal on physical exam, and not interfering with function	mild symptoms interfering with function but not interfering with activities of daily living	moderate symptoms interfering with activities of daily living	bedridden or disabling
CNS cerebrovascular ischemia	none	-	-	transient ischemic event or attack (TIA)	permanent event (e.g., cerebral vascular accident)

CNS hemorrhage/bleeding is graded in the HEMORRHAGE category.

Adverse Event	0	1	2	3	4
Cognitive disturbance/learning problems	*none*	*cognitive disability; not interfering with work/ school performance; preservation of intelligence*	*cognitive disability; interfering with work/ school performance; decline of 1 SD (Standard Deviation) or loss of developmental milestones*	*cognitive disability; resulting in significant impairment of work/ school performance; cognitive decline > 2 SD*	*inability to work/ frank mental retardation*

(Continued on next page)

Adverse Event	Grade 0	1	2	3	4
Confusion	normal	confusion or disorientation or attention deficit of brief duration; resolves spontaneously with no sequelae	confusion or disorientation or attention deficit interfering with function, but not interfering with activities of daily living	confusion or delirium interfering with activities of daily living	harmful to others or self; requiring hospitalization

Cranial neuropathy is graded in the NEUROLOGY category as Neuropathy-cranial.

Adverse Event	0	1	2	3	4
Delusions	normal	-	-	present	toxic psychosis
Depressed level of consciousness	normal	somnolence or sedation not interfering with function	somnolence or sedation interfering with function, but not interfering with activities of daily living	obtundation or stupor; difficult to arouse; interfering with activities of daily living	coma

Syncope (fainting) is graded in the NEUROLOGY category.

Adverse Event	0	1	2	3	4
Dizziness/ lightheadedness	none	not interfering with function	interfering with function, but not interfering with activities of daily living	interfering with activities of daily living	bedridden or disabling

Dysphasia, receptive and/or expressive, is graded under Speech impairment in the NEUROLOGY category.

Adverse Event	0	1	2	3	4
Extrapyramidal/ involuntary movement/ restlessness	none	mild involuntary movements not interfering with function	moderate involuntary movements interfering with function, but not interfering with activities of daily living	severe involuntary movements or torticollis interfering with activities of daily living	bedridden or disabling
Hallucinations	normal	-	-	present	toxic psychosis

Headache is graded in the PAIN category.

Adverse Event	0	1	2	3	4
Insomnia	normal	occasional difficulty sleeping not interfering with function	difficulty sleeping interfering with function, but not interfering with activities of daily living	frequent difficulty sleeping, interfering with activities of daily living	-

Note: This adverse event is graded when insomnia is related to treatment. If pain or other symptoms interfere with sleep, do NOT grade as insomnia.

Adverse Event	0	1	2	3	4
Irritability (children < 3 years of age)	*normal*	*mild; easily consolable*	*moderate; requiring increased attention*	*severe; inconsolable*	*-*
Leukoencephalopathy associated radiological findings	none	mild increase in SAS (subarachnoid space) and/or mild ventriculomegaly; and/or small (+/- multiple) focal T2 hyperintensities, involving periventricular white matter or < 1/3 of susceptible areas of cerebrum	moderate increase in SAS; and/or moderate ventriculomegaly; and/or focal T2 hyperintensities extending into centrum ovale; or involving 1/3 to 2/3 of susceptible areas of cerebrum	severe increase in SAS; severe ventriculomegaly; near total white matter T2 hyperintensities or diffuse low attenuation (CT); focal white matter necrosis (cystic)	severe increase in SAS; severe ventriculomegaly; diffuse low attenuation with calcification (CT); diffuse white matter necrosis (MRI)
Memory loss	normal	memory loss not interfering with function	memory loss interfering with function, but not interfering with activities of daily living	memory loss interfering with activities of daily living	amnesia
Mood alteration— anxiety, agitation	normal		mild mood alteration not interfering with function moderate mood alteration interfering	with function, but not interfering with activities of daily living severe mood	alteration interfering with activities of daily living suicidal ideation or danger to self

(Continued on next page)

APPENDICES

Appendix 1. National Cancer Institute Common Toxicity Criteria (CTC) *(Continued)*

Adverse Event	0	1	2	3	4
			Grade		
Mood alteration—depression	normal	mild mood alteration not interfering with function	moderate mood alteration interfering with function, but not interfering with activities of daily living	severe mood alteration interfering with activities of daily living	suicidal ideation or danger to self
Mood alteration—euphoria	normal	mild mood alteration not interfering with function	moderate mood alteration interfering with function, but not interfering with activities of daily living	severe mood alteration interfering with activities of daily living	danger to self
Neuropathic pain is graded in the PAIN category.					
Neuropathy—cranial	absent	-	present, not interfering with activities of daily living	present, interfering with activities of daily living	life-threatening, disabling
Neuropathy—motor	normal	subjective weakness but no objective findings	mild objective weakness interfering with function, but not interfering with activities of daily living	objective weakness interfering with activities of daily living	paralysis
Neuropathy—sensory	normal	loss of deep tendon reflexes or paresthesia (including tingling), but not interfering with function	objective sensory loss or paresthesia (including tingling), interfering with function, but not interfering with activities of daily living	sensory loss or paresthesia interfering with activities of daily living permanent sensory	loss that interferes with function
Nystagmus *Also consider Vision—double vision.*	absent	present	-	-	-
Personality/behavioral	normal	change, but not disruptive to patient or family	disruptive to patient or family	disruptive to patient and family; requiring mental health intervention	harmful to others or self; requiring hospitalization
Pyramidal tract dysfunction (e.g., tone, hyperreflexia, positive Babinski, fine motor coordination)	normal	asymptomatic with abnormality on physical examination	symptomatic or interfering with function, but not interfering with activities of daily living	interfering with activities of daily living	bedridden or disabling; paralysis
Seizure(s)	none	-	seizure(s) self-limited and consciousness is preserved	seizure(s) in which consciousness is altered	seizures of any type that are prolonged, repetitive, or difficult to control (e.g., status epilepticus, intractable epilepsy)
Speech impairment (e.g., dysphasia or aphasia)	normal	-	awareness of receptive or expressive dysphasia, not impairing ability to communicate	receptive or expressive dysphasia, impairing ability to communicate	inability to communicate
Syncope (fainting) *Also consider CARDIOVASCULAR (ARRHYTHMIA), Vasovagal episode, CNS cerebrovascular ischemia.*	absent	-	-	present	-
Tremor	none	mild and brief or intermittent but not interfering with function	moderate tremor interfering with function, but not interfering with activities of daily living	severe tremor interfering with activities of daily living	-

(Continued on next page)

Adverse Event	Grade 0	Grade 1	Grade 2	Grade 3	Grade 4
Vertigo	none	not interfering with function	interfering with function, but not interfering with activities of daily living	interfering with activities of daily living	bedridden or disabling
Neurology-Other (Specify, _____)	none	mild	moderate	severe	life-threatening or disabling

OCULAR/VISUAL

Adverse Event	Grade 0	Grade 1	Grade 2	Grade 3	Grade 4
Cataract	none	asymptomatic	symptomatic, partial visual loss	symptomatic, visual loss requiring treatment or interfering with function	-
Conjunctivitis	none	abnormal ophthalmologic changes, but asymptomatic or symptomatic without visual impairment (i.e., pain and irritation)	symptomatic and interfering with function, but not interfering with activities of daily living	symptomatic and interfering with activities of daily living	-
Dry eye	none	mild, not requiring treatment	moderate or requiring artificial tears	-	-
Glaucoma	none	increase in intraocular pressure but no visual loss	increase in intraocular pressure with retinal changes	visual impairment	unilateral or bilateral loss of vision (blindness)
Keratitis (corneal inflammation/corneal ulceration)	none	abnormal ophthalmologic changes but asymptomatic or symptomatic without visual impairment (i.e., pain and irritation)	symptomatic and interfering with function, but not interfering with activities of daily living	symptomatic and interfering with activities of daily living	unilateral or bilateral loss of vision (blindness)
Tearing (watery eyes)	none	mild, not interfering with function	moderate: interfering with function, but not interfering with activities of daily living	interfering with activities of daily living	-
Vision—blurred vision	none	-	symptomatic and interfering with function, but not interfering with activities of daily living	symptomatic and interfering with activities of daily living	-
Vision—double vision (diplopia)	normal	-	symptomatic and interfering with function, but not interfering with activities of daily living	symptomatic and interfering with activities of daily living	-
Vision—flashing lights/floaters	normal	mild, not interfering with function	symptomatic and interfering with function, but not interfering with activities of daily living	symptomatic and interfering with activities of daily living	-
Vision—night blindness (nyctalopia)	normal	abnormal electro-retinography but asymptomatic	symptomatic and interfering with function, but not interfering with activities of daily living	symptomatic and interfering with activities of daily living	-
Vision—photophobia	normal	-	symptomatic and interfering with function, but not interfering with activities of daily living	symptomatic and interfering with activities of daily living	-
Ocular/Visual-Other (Specify, _____)	normal	mild	moderate	severe	unilateral or bilateral loss of vision (blindness)

(Continued on next page)

APPENDICES

Adverse Event	0	1	Grade 2	3	4

PAIN

Adverse Event	0	1	2	3	4
Abdominal pain or cramping	none	mild pain not interfering with function	moderate pain: pain or analgesics interfering with function, but not interfering with activities of daily living	severe pain: pain or analgesics severely interfering with activities of daily living	disabling
Arthralgia (joint pain)	none	mild pain not interfering with function	moderate pain: pain or analgesics interfering with function, but not interfering with activities of daily living	severe pain: pain or analgesics severely interfering with activities of daily living	disabling

Arthritis (joint pain with clinical signs of inflammation) is graded in the MUSCULOSKELETAL category.

Adverse Event	0	1	2	3	4
Bone pain	none	mild pain not interfering with function	moderate pain: pain or analgesics interfering with function, but not interfering with activities of daily living	severe pain: pain or analgesics severely interfering with activities of daily living	disabling
Chest pain (non-cardiac and non-pleuritic)	none	mild pain not interfering with function	moderate pain: pain or analgesics interfering with function, but not interfering with activities of daily living	severe pain: pain or analgesics severely interfering with activities of daily living	disabling
Dysmenorrhea	none	mild pain not interfering with function	moderate pain: pain or analgesics interfering with function, but not interfering with activities of daily living	severe pain: pain or analgesics severely interfering with activities of daily living	disabling
Dyspareunia	none	mild pain not interfering with function	moderate pain interfering with sexual activity	severe pain preventing sexual activity	-

Dysuria is graded in the RENAL/GENITOURINARY category.

Adverse Event	0	1	2	3	4
Earache (otalgia)	none	mild pain not interfering with function	moderate pain: pain or analgesics interfering with function, but not interfering with activities of daily living	severe pain: pain or analgesics severely interfering with activities of daily living	disabling
Headache	none	mild pain not interfering with function	moderate pain: pain or analgesics interfering with function, but not interfering with activities of daily living	severe pain: pain or analgesics severely interfering with activities of daily living	disabling
Hepatic pain	none	mild pain not interfering with function	moderate pain: pain or analgesics interfering with function, but not interfering with activities of daily living	severe pain: pain or analgesics severely interfering with activities of daily living	disabling
Myalgia (muscle pain)	none	mild pain not interfering with function	moderate pain: pain or analgesics interfering with function, but not interfering with activities of daily living	severe pain: pain or analgesics severely interfering with activities of daily living	disabling
Neuropathic pain (e.g., jaw pain, neurologic pain, phantom limb pain, post infectious neuralgia, or painful neuropathies)	none	mild pain not interfering with function	moderate pain: pain or analgesics interfering with function, but not interfering with activities of daily living	severe pain: pain or analgesics severely interfering with activities of daily living	disabling

(Continued on next page)

APPENDICES

Appendix 1. National Cancer Institute Common Toxicity Criteria (CTC) *(Continued)*

Adverse Event	Grade 0	1	2	3	4
Pain due to radiation	none	mild pain not interfering with function	moderate pain: pain or analgesics interfering with function, but not interfering with activities of daily living	severe pain: pain or analgesics severely interfering with activities of daily living	disabling
Pelvic pain	none	mild pain not interfering with function	moderate pain: pain or analgesics interfering with function, but not interfering with activities of daily living	severe pain: pain or analgesics severely interfering with activities of daily living	disabling
Pleuritic pain	none	mild pain not interfering with function	moderate pain: pain or analgesics interfering with function, but not interfering with activities of daily living	severe pain: pain or analgesics severely interfering with activities of daily living	disabling
Rectal or perirectal pain (proctalgia)	none	mild pain not interfering with function	moderate pain: pain or analgesics interfering with function, but not interfering with activities of daily living	severe pain: pain or analgesics severely interfering with activities of daily living	disabling
Tumor pain (onset or exacerbation of tumor pain due to treatment)	none	mild pain not interfering with function	moderate pain: pain or analgesics interfering with function, but not interfering with activities of daily living	severe pain: pain or analgesics severely interfering with activities of daily living	disabling
Tumor flare is graded in the SYNDROME category.					
Pain-Other (Specify, _____)	none	mild	moderate	severe	disabling
PULMONARY					
Adult Respiratory Distress Syndrome (ARDS)	absent	-	-	-	present
Apnea	none	-	-	present	requiring intubation
Carbon monoxide diffusion capacity (DL$_{CO}$)	≥ 90% of pretreatment or normal value	≥ 75–< 90% of pretreatment or normal value	≥ 50–< 75% of pretreatment or normal value	≥ 25–< 50% of pretreatment or normal value	< 25% of pretreatment or normal value
Cough	absent	mild, relieved by non-prescription medication	requiring narcotic antitussive	severe cough or coughing spasms, poorly controlled or unresponsive to treatment	-
Dyspnea (shortness of breath)	normal	-	dyspnea on exertion	dyspnea at normal level of activity	dyspnea at rest or requiring ventilator support
Forced Expiratory Volume (FEV$_1$)	≥ 90% of pretreatment or normal value	≥ 75–< 90% of pretreatment or normal value	≥ 50–< 75% of pretreatment or normal value	≥ 25–< 50% of pretreatment or normal value	< 25% of pretreatment or normal value
Hiccoughs (hiccups, singultus)	none	mild, not requiring treatment	moderate, requiring treatment	severe, prolonged, and refractory to treatment	-

(Continued on next page)

Appendix 1. National Cancer Institute Common Toxicity Criteria (CTC) *(Continued)*

Adverse Event	0	1	2	3	4
			Grade		
Hypoxia	normal	-	decreased O$_2$ saturation with exercise	decreased O$_2$ saturation at rest, requiring supplemental oxygen	decreased O$_2$ saturation, requiring pressure support (CPAP) or assisted ventilation
Pleural effusion (non-malignant)	none	asymptomatic and not requiring treatment	symptomatic, requiring diuretics	symptomatic, requiring O$_2$ or therapeutic thoracentesis	life-threatening (e.g., requiring intubation)
Pleuritic pain is graded in the PAIN category.					
Pneumonitis/pulmonary infiltrates	none	radiographic changes but asymptomatic or symptoms not requiring steroids	radiographic changes and requiring steroids or diuretics	radiographic changes and requiring oxygen	radiographic changes and requiring assisted ventilation
Pneumothorax	none	no intervention required	chest tube required	sclerosis or surgery required	life-threatening
Pulmonary embolism is graded as Thrombosis/embolism in the CARDIOVASCULAR (GENERAL) category.					
Pulmonary fibrosis	none	radiographic changes, but asymptomatic or symptoms not requiring steroids	requiring steroids or diuretics	requiring oxygen	requiring assisted ventilation
Radiation-related pulmonary fibrosis is graded in the RTOG/EORTC Late Radiation Morbidity Scoring Scheme—Lung.					
Voice changes/stridor/larynx (e.g., hoarseness, loss of voice, laryngitis)	normal	mild or intermittent hoarseness	persistent hoarseness, but able to vocalize; may have mild to moderate edema	whispered speech, not able to vocalize; may have marked edema	marked dyspnea/stridor requiring tracheostomy or intubation
Notes: Cough from radiation is graded as cough in the PULMONARY category.					
Radiation-related hemoptysis from larynx/pharynx is graded as Grade 4 Mucositis due to radiation in the GASTROINTESTINAL category. Radiation-related hemoptysis from the thoracic cavity is graded as Grade 4 Hemoptysis in the HEMORRHAGE category.					
Pulmonary-Other (Specify, _____)	none	mild	moderate	severe	life-threatening or disabling
RENAL/GENITOURINARY					
Bladder spasms	absent	mild symptoms, not requiring intervention	symptoms requiring antispasmodic	severe symptoms requiring narcotic	-
Creatinine	WNL	> ULN–1.5 x ULN	> 1.5–3.0 x ULN	> 3.0–6.0 x ULN	> 6.0 x ULN
Note: Adjust to age-appropriate levels for pediatric patients.					
Dysuria (painful urination)	none	mild symptoms requiring no intervention	symptoms relieved with therapy	symptoms not relieved despite therapy	-
Fistula or GU fistula (e.g., vaginal, vesico-vaginal)	none	-	-	requiring intervention	requiring surgery
Hemoglobinuria	-	present	-	-	-
Hematuria (in the absence of vaginal bleeding) is graded in the HEMORRHAGE category.					
Incontinence	none	with coughing, sneezing, etc.	spontaneous, some control	no control (in the absence of fistula)	-
Operative injury to bladder and/or ureter	none	-	injury of bladder with primary repair	sepsis, fistula, or obstruction requiring secondary surgery; loss of one kidney; injury requiring anastomosis or reimplantation	septic obstruction of both kidneys or vesicovaginal fistula requiring diversion

(Continued on next page)

Adverse Event	0	1	2	3	4
			Grade		
Proteinuria	normal or < 0.15 g/24 hours	1+ or 0.15 1.0 g/24 hours	2+ to 3+ or 1.0 3.5 g/ 24 hours	4+ or > 3.5 g/24 hours	nephrotic syndrome

Note: If there is an inconsistency between absolute value and dip stick reading, use the absolute value for grading.

Adverse Event	0	1	2	3	4
Renal failure	none	-	-	requiring dialysis, but reversible	requiring dialysis and irreversible
Ureteral obstruction	none	unilateral, not requiring surgery	-	bilateral, not requiring surgery	stent, nephrostomy tube, or surgery
Urinary electrolyte wasting (e.g., Fanconi's syndrome, renal tubular acidosis)	none	asymptomatic, not requiring treatment	mild, reversible, and manageable with oral replacement	reversible but requiring IV replace- ment	irreversible, requiring continued replacement

Also consider Acidosis, Bicarbonate, Hypocalcemia, Hypophosphatemia.

Adverse Event	0	1	2	3	4
Urinary frequency/ urgency	normal	increase in frequency or nocturia up to 2 x normal	increase > 2 x normal but < hourly	hourly or more with urgency, or requiring catheter	-
Urinary retention	normal	hesitancy or dribbling, but no significant re- sidual urine; retention occurring during the immediate postop- erative period	hesitancy requiring medication or occa- sional in/out catheter- ization (< 4 x per week), or operative bladder atony requiring indwelling catheter be- yond immediate post- operative period but for < 6 weeks	requiring frequent in/ out catheterization (≥ 4 x per week) or urological intervention (e.g., TURP, suprapu- bic tube, urethrotomy)	bladder rupture
Urine color change (not related to other dietary or physi- ologic cause e.g., bilirubin, concen- trated urine, hem- aturia)	normal	asymptomatic, change in urine color	-	-	-

Vaginal bleeding is graded in the HEMORRHAGE category.

Adverse Event	0	1	2	3	4
Vaginitis (not due to infection)	none	mild, not requiring treatment	moderate, relieved with treatment	severe, not relieved with treatment, or ulceration not requiring surgery	ulceration requiring surgery
Renal/Genitouri- nary-Other (Specify, _____)	none	mild	moderate	severe	life-threatening or disabling

SECONDARY MALIGNANCY

Adverse Event	0	1	2	3	4
Secondary Malignancy-Other (Specify type, _____) excludes metasta- sis from initial primary.	none	-	-	-	present

SEXUAL/REPRODUCTIVE FUNCTION

Dyspareunia is graded in the PAIN category.

Dysmenorrhea is graded in the PAIN category.

Adverse Event	0	1	2	3	4
Erectile impotence	normal	mild (erections impaired but satisfac- tory)	moderate (erections impaired, unsatisfac- tory for intercourse)	no erections	-

(Continued on next page)

APPENDICES

Toxicity	Grade				
	0	1	2	3	4
Female sterility	normal	-	-	sterile	-
Feminization of male is graded in the ENDOCRINE category.					
Irregular menses (change from baseline)	normal	occasionally irregular or lengthened interval, but continuing menstrual cycles	very irregular, but continuing menstrual cycles	persistent amenorrhea	-
Libido	normal	decrease in interest	severe loss of interest	-	-
Male infertility	-	-	oligospermia (low sperm count)	azoospermia (no sperm)	-
Masculinization of female is graded in the ENDOCRINE category.					
Vaginal dryness	normal	mild	requiring treatment and/or interfering with sexual function, dyspareunia	-	-
Sexual/Reproductive Function-Other (Specify, _____)	none	mild	moderate	severe	disabling

SYNDROMES (not included in previous categories)

Acute vascular leak syndrome is graded in the CARDIOVASCULAR (GENERAL) category.

ARDS (Adult Respiratory Distress Syndrome) is graded in the PULMONARY category.

Autoimmune reactions are graded in the ALLERGY/IMMUNOLOGY category.

DIC (disseminated intravascular coagulation) is graded in the COAGULATION category.

Fanconi's syndrome is graded as Urinary electrolyte wasting in the RENAL/GENITOURINARY category.

Renal tubular acidosis is graded as Urinary electrolyte wasting in the RENAL/GENITOURINARY category.

Stevens-Johnson syndrome (erythema multiforme) is graded in the DERMATOLOGY/SKIN category.

SIADH (syndrome of inappropriate antidiuretic hormone) is graded in the ENDOCRINE category.

Thrombotic microangiopathy (e.g., thrombotic thrombocytopenic purpura/TTP or hemolytic uremic syndrome/HUS) is graded in the COAGULATION category.

Toxicity	0	1	2	3	4
Tumor flare	none	mild pain not interfering with function	moderate pain; pain or analgesics interfering with function, but not interfering with activities of daily living	severe pain; pain or analgesics interfering with function and interfering with activities of daily living	disabling

Also consider Hypercalcemia.

Note: Tumor flare is characterized by a constellation of symptoms and signs in direct relation to initiation of therapy (e.g., antiestrogens/androgens or additional hormones). The symptoms/signs include tumor pain, inflammation of visible tumor, hypercalcemia, diffuse bone pain, and other electrolyte disturbances.

Toxicity	0	1	2	3	4
Tumor lysis syndrome	absent	-	-	present	-

Also consider Hyperkalemia, Creatinine.

Urinary electrolyte wasting (e.g., Fanconi's syndrome, renal tubular acidosis) is graded under the RENAL/GENITOURINARY category.

Toxicity	0	1	2	3	4
Syndromes-Other (Specify, _____)	none	mild	moderate	severe	life-threatening or disabling

Note. From *National Cancer Institute Common Toxicity Criteria, Version 2.0* [Online], revised March 23, 1998. Available: http://ctep.info.nih.gov/CTC3/ctc.htm [1999, January 20].

Appendix 2. Safe Management of Chemotherapy in the Home

You are receiving chemotherapy to treat or control your cancer. In the past few years, people with cancer have been able to receive these drugs in the ambulatory oncology setting, the hospital, or at home. Chemotherapy can be administered by injection, intravenously, or orally. Its purpose is to kill or stop cancer cells from growing, but it also may damage normal cells. Special precautions must be taken to prevent chemotherapy from coming into accidental contact with you or others. This pamphlet teaches you and your family how to avoid exposure to chemotherapy and how to handle hazardous waste in your home.

Chemotherapy Is Hazardous Waste

Chemotherapy medicine, equipment, or items that come into contact with the medicine (i.e., syringes, needles) at any time are considered contaminated with hazardous waste. Regardless of its administration method, chemotherapy remains in your body for many hours, sometimes days, after your treatment and is excreted in urine and stool. If you are vomiting, the vomitus may contain traces of chemotherapy.

Hazardous Waste Disposal

Chemotherapy is considered hazardous waste. Materials contaminated with chemotherapy must be disposed of in specially marked containers. You will be given a hard plastic container labeled "Chemotherapy" or "Hazardous Waste." Equipment and gloves that have been in contact with chemotherapy should be placed into this container. If materials in contact with chemotherapy are too large to fit in the plastic container, place them in a special bag and seal it tightly with rubber bands. Sharp objects should only be placed in hard plastic containers. Ask your doctor or nurse which containers you should use. Containers or bags should be removed from your home when full. Either return waste containers to your physician's office or arrange for the company supplying your medicines and equipment to remove the waste.

Body Wastes

You may use the toilet (septic tank or city sewage) as usual, just flush it twice after using for 48 hours after receiving chemotherapy. Wash your hands well with soap and water afterward, and wash your skin if urine or stool gets on it. Pregnant women should avoid direct contact with chemotherapy or contaminated wastes.

Laundry

Items soiled with chemotherapy should be handled carefully to avoid getting the drug on your skin. Wear gloves to immediately place soiled sheets and clothing in the washer and wash as usual. If you do not have a washer, place soiled items in a plastic bag until they can be washed. Wash unsoiled clothes and linens in the usual manner. Also, dispose of plastic sheets as hazardous waste.

Skin Care

Chemotherapy spilled on the skin may cause irritation. If this happens, thoroughly wash the area with soap and water, then dry. If redness persists more than one hour or if irritation occurs, call your doctor. Because chemotherapy is absorbed through the skin, gloves should be worn when working with the chemotherapy, equipment, or wastes.

Eye Care

If any chemotherapy splashes into your eyes, flush them out with water for 10–15 minutes and notify your doctor.

QUESTIONS AND ANSWERS

Is it safe for family members to have contact with me during my chemotherapy?

Yes. Being with your loved ones is an important part of life. Eating together, enjoying favorite activities, hugging, and kissing are all safe.

Is it safe for my family to use the same toilet as I do?

Yes. As long as any chemotherapy waste is cleaned from the toilet, sharing is safe.

What should I do if I do not have control of my bladder or bowels?

Use a disposable, plastic-backed pad, diaper, or sheet to absorb urine or stool. Change immediately when soiled and wash skin with soap and water. If you have an ostomy, your caregiver should wear gloves when emptying or changing appliances. Used ostomy supplies must be handled as hazardous waste.

What if I use a bedpan, urinal, or commode?

Your caregiver should wear gloves when emptying the wastes. Rinse the container with water after each use, and wash it with soap and water at least once a day.

What if I vomit?

Your caregiver should wear gloves when emptying the basin. Rinse it with water after each use. Wash the basin at least once a day with soap and water.

Is if safe to be sexually active during my treatment?

Most often, yes. Special precautions may need to be taken (ask your doctor or nurse). Chemotherapy is present in urine, stool, and vomitus, and it is probable that traces of chemotherapy are present in vaginal fluid and semen.

Is it possible to become pregnant or father a child while receiving chemotherapy?

Yes. A reliable method of birth control should be used while you are receiving chemotherapy.

How should I store chemotherapy at home?

Chemotherapy and equipment should be stored in a safe place, out of reach of children and pets. Do not store chemotherapy in the bathroom, as high humidity may damage the drugs. Check medicine labels to see if your chemotherapy should be kept in the refrigerator or away from light, and be sure all medicines are completely labeled.

Is it safe to dispose of chemotherapy in the trash?

No. Chemotherapy is hazardous waste that should be handled separately. If you are administering IV chemotherapy at home, you should have a special container in which to put all chemotherapy and equipment. This includes used syringes, needles, tubing, bags, cassettes, and vials. This container should be hard plastic and labeled "Hazardous Waste" or "Biohazard." Normally, you will not have extra oral chemotherapy medicine, but if you do, return it to your doctor or nurse for disposal. *Do not throw any hazardous wastes into the garbage!*

Can I travel with my chemotherapy?

Yes. Usually, traveling is no problem. However, because some chemotherapy requires special storage (e.g., refrigeration), you may need to make special arrangements. Check with your nurse, doctor, or medicine supplier for further instructions. Regardless of your means of travel (airplanes, cars, etc.), always seal your chemotherapy drugs in a plastic bag.

What should I do if I spill some chemotherapy?

In the event of a chemotherapy spill, clean the area wearing two pairs of gloves, a mask, gown, and goggles. Absorb the spill with a disposable sponge. Clean the area with soap and water. Dispose of materials in the chemotherapy hazardous waste container.

Note. From "Safe Management of Chemotherapy at Home," by G. Sansivero and S. Murray, 1989, *Oncology Nursing Forum, 16*(5), pp. 711–713. Copyright 1989 by the Oncology Nursing Press, Inc. Adapted with permission.

APPENDICES

Appendix 3. Nursing Flow Sheet[a]

Name _____ Age _____ Diagnosis _____

Allergies _____

Medical Problems _____

Date					
RN signature					
Type of visit P/C					
VAD P/H					
VAD flush					
Comments					
Vesicant location 1–5 R/L					
Reactions					
Mucositis 0–3					
Infection specify					
Rx					
Resolved					
Alopecia 0–3					
Scalp hypothermia Y/N					
Bleeding Y/N					
Comments					
Diarrhea # episodes/24 hours					
Rx					
Constipation # BM/qd/qwk					
Normal/Abnormal N/ABNL					
Rx					
Bladder symptoms 0–5					
Rx					
Relief Y/N					
Pain Y/N					
Sites					
Intensity 0–10					
Characteristics C/I					
Analgesics					
Relief 0–10					
Relief adequate Y/N					
Comments					

[a] As used at New Haven Hospital, New Haven, CT

(Continued on next page)

Date				
Insomnia Y/N				
Rx				
Rx effective Y/N				
Fatigue 0–10				
Nausea severity 0–3				
Vomiting # episodes/24 hours				
Duration				
Antiemetic relief 1,2				
Comments				
Appetite 0–4				
Diet 1–5				
Supplements, amount/24 hours				
Altered taste Y/N				
Other				
Cough Y/N				
Productive Y/N				
Rx				
Relief 1,2				
SOB 0–3				
O_2 specify				
Sexual difficulties 0–3				
Mobility 1–4				
Motor weakness 0–3				
Neuropathy 0–3				
Comments				
Anxiety 0–3				
Coping effectiveness Y/N				
Rx				
Counseling Y/N				
Homecare agency (specify)				
VNA/hospice				
HHA/homemaker				
Social services				
Patient education 1–7				
Education materials				
Other				

(Continued on next page)

APPENDICES

Nursing Flow Sheet Key

Date	
RN signature	
Type of visit	P = Phone C = Clinic
VAD	P = Port H = Hickman
VAD flush	Check, specify heparin amount
Comments	Note difficulty drawing blood, etc.

Vesicant location   1–5, see diagram   R = right / L = left

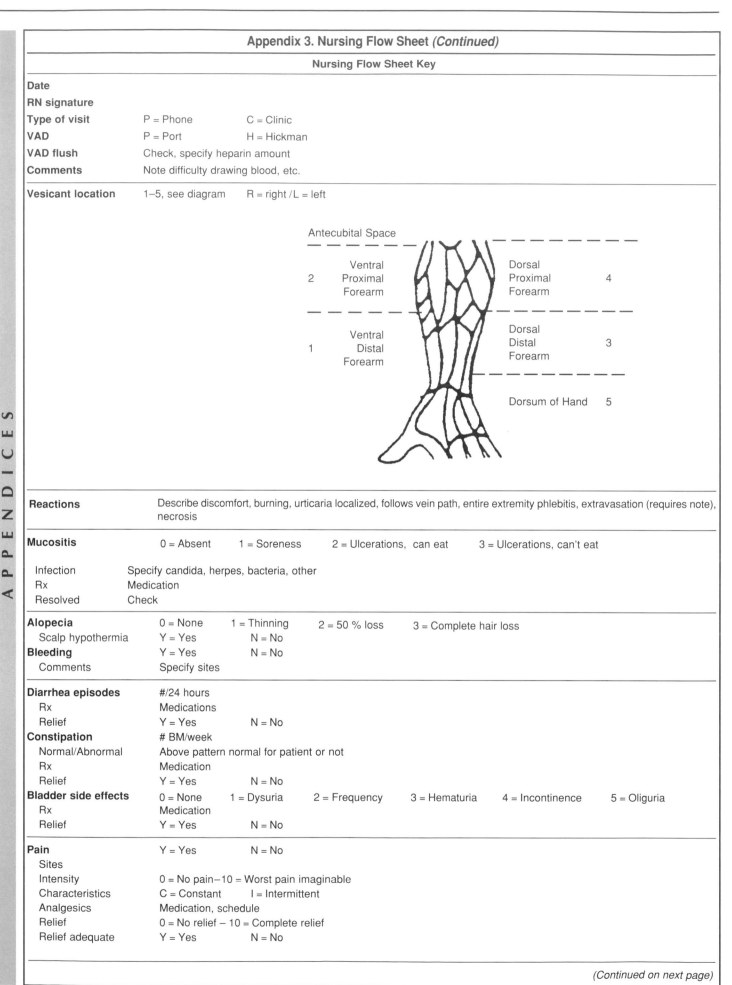

Antecubital Space

2 Ventral Proximal Forearm   Dorsal Proximal Forearm 4

1 Ventral Distal Forearm   Dorsal Distal Forearm 3

Dorsum of Hand 5

Reactions	Describe discomfort, burning, urticaria localized, follows vein path, entire extremity phlebitis, extravasation (requires note), necrosis

Mucositis   0 = Absent   1 = Soreness   2 = Ulcerations, can eat   3 = Ulcerations, can't eat

Infection	Specify candida, herpes, bacteria, other
Rx	Medication
Resolved	Check

Alopecia   0 = None   1 = Thinning   2 = 50 % loss   3 = Complete hair loss

Scalp hypothermia	Y = Yes N = No
Bleeding	Y = Yes N = No
Comments	Specify sites

Diarrhea episodes	#/24 hours
Rx	Medications
Relief	Y = Yes N = No
Constipation	# BM/week
Normal/Abnormal	Above pattern normal for patient or not
Rx	Medication
Relief	Y = Yes N = No

Bladder side effects   0 = None   1 = Dysuria   2 = Frequency   3 = Hematuria   4 = Incontinence   5 = Oliguria

Rx	Medication
Relief	Y = Yes N = No

Pain	Y = Yes N = No
Sites	
Intensity	0 = No pain–10 = Worst pain imaginable
Characteristics	C = Constant I = Intermittent
Analgesics	Medication, schedule
Relief	0 = No relief – 10 = Complete relief
Relief adequate	Y = Yes N = No

(Continued on next page)

APPENDICES

Appendix 3. Nursing Flow Sheet *(Continued)*

Nursing Flow Sheet Key

Insomnia	Y = Yes	N = No			
Rx	Medication				
Rx effective	Y = Yes	N = No			
Fatigue	0 = Quite rested	−10 = Completely exhausted			

Nausea severity	0 = None	1 = Mild	2 = Moderate	3 = Severe	
Vomiting episodes	# vomiting episodes/24 hrs.				
Duration	# hrs. after chemo vomiting started/stopped (e.g.,+3/+18)				
Antiemetic relief	1 = Adequate	2 = Inadequate			
Comments					

Appetite	0 = None	1 = 25% normal	2 = 50% normal	3 = 75% normal	4 = 100%
Diet	1 = Solids	2 = Liquids	3 = Soft	4 = 1,2 + supplements	5 = Supplements
Supplements	Specify type and amount/24 hrs				
Altered taste	Y = Yes	N = No			
Comments					

Cough	Y = Yes	N = No		
Productive	Y = Yes	N = No		
Rx	Medication			
Relief	1 = Adequate	2 = Inadequate		
SOB	0 = None	1 = Mild	2 = Moderate	3 – Severe
O$_2$	Specify liter flow			

Sexual difficulties	0 = None	1 = Mild dysfunction	2 = Moderate dysfunction	3 = Severe limitations

Mobility	1 = Ambulatory	2 = Ambulatory with assist	3 = Wheel chair	4 = Bedridden
Motor weakness	0 = None	1 = Mild	2 = Moderate	3 = Severe
Neuropathy	0 = None	1 = Paresthesias, numbness/tingling feet and/or fingers	2 = Slapping gait, ataxia	3 = Visual, auditory disturbances
Comments	Location, etiology of muscle weakness, etc.			

Anxiety	0 = None	1 = Mild	2 = Moderate	3 = Severe
Coping effectiveness	Y = Yes	N = No		
Rx	Medication			
Counseling	Y = Yes	N = No		

Home care agency	Specify name of agency, date initiated and discharged
VNA/hospice	Check
HHA/homemaker	Check, note hrs./day or week
Social services	Check

Patient education	1 = Chemo side effects	2 = Symptom management	3 = Emergency phone number	4 = Home care resources	5 = Community	6 = Coping	7 = Specify
Education materials	Pamphlets or brochures given, videos used, etc.						

Other	e.g., complaints, problems, appliances (ostomies, trach, etc.)

Note. From "A Nursing Flow Sheet for Documentation of Ambulatory Oncology," by J.M. Moore and M.T. Knobf, 1991, *Oncology Nursing Forum, 18,* pp. 934–937. Copyright 1991 by Oncology Nursing Press, Inc. Reprinted with permission.

APPENDICES

Appendix 4. Chemotherapy Flow Sheet[a]

RX: Anti-Tumor Drugs & Dose (Meds, RT, etc.)							
Date							
Day on study							
Course							
Dose ADJ/CD							
Transfusion							

Symptoms							
Performance							
Pain							
Food intake							
Vomiting							
Diarrhea/constipation							
Bleeding							
Mucosa							
Respiratory							
Urinary							
CNS							
Weight							

Physical Findings							
Temperature/respiration							
Blood pressure/pulse							
Skin / mouth							
Breast / nodes							
Chest							
Heart							
Abdomen							
Liver / spleen							
Neurologic							
Rectal							
Status							

Tumor Measurement							
1.							
2.							
3.							
4.							

Laboratory							
WBC							
Granulocyte							
Lymphocytes							
Monocytes							
HGB HCT							
Retics							
Platelets							
BUN CREAT							
Uric AC CA++							
SGOT LDH							
ALKP'TASE							
BILI T/D							
CEA							
Radiology							
Initials							

Study _____ MR# _____

DX _____

Page _____ of Study _____

Continue remarks on reverse

Age _____

Height _____

M^2 _____

[a] As used at Deaconess Hospital in Boston, MA

(Continued on next page)

Appendix 4. Chemotherapy Flow Sheet *(Continued)*

Administration						
	Date					
	IV site					
	Needle type and size					
	Adverse reactions					
	Treatment schedule: drug and administration method					

Patient Teaching						
	Instructions per institutional instruction sheets for:					
	Self-care measures per institutional standards of care for:					
	Nausea / vomiting					
	Myelosuppression					
	Mouth care					

Nursing Observations/Assessments/Management						
	Acknowledgement of initial teaching (patient signature)					
	Nurse:					

I = Initial teaching   R = Reviewed   W = Written materials given   P = See progress note   N/A = Not applicable   S = Side effects verbalized or reported

Key								
	RN			RN		RN		RN
	RN			RN		RN		RN

Note. From "Flowsheet Documentation of Chemotherapy Administration and Patient Teaching," by M. Lynch and L. Yanes, 1991, *Oncology Nursing Forum 18*, pp. 777–783. Copyright 1991 by Oncology Nursing Press, Inc. Adapted with permission.

APPENDICES

Appendix 5. Clinical Practicum Evaluation: Part I

As part of the nurse's evaluation, the preceptor will verify performance of basic skills by indicating whether the nurse completes the following.

	Yes	No	NA
1. Checks appropriate laboratory data prior to reconstituting chemotherapy			
2. Verifies physician's written order for specific dosage, route, and mode of administration			
3. Calculates drug dosage based on patient's height and weight			
4. Observes precautions in drug preparation and handling			
5. Maintains aseptic technique			
6. Reconstitutes drugs under sterile conditions according to the package insert			
7. Discards unused portion of drug in proper container			
8. Takes appropriate action in the event of drug spillage			
9. Takes appropriate action in the event of drug spray or contact with skin or mucous membranes			
10. Correctly labels drug with patient's name, room number, drug name, drug dose and amount per unit volume, route of administration, date and time prepared, vesicant, and storage requirements			
11. Verifies drug dosage a second time			
12. Correctly states immediate and delayed side effects of the drugs			
13. Assures patient identification			
14. Identifies self to patient			
15. Informs patient of procedure for reaching a nurse during treatment			
16. Reviews patient's allergy history			
17. Verifies that informed consent has occurred, if investigational protocol			
18. Ensures patient comfort and provides antiemetic if indicated			
19. Explains procedure and any side effects of the drugs and answers patient's questions appropriately			
20. Assesses patient's response to previous therapy			
21. Teaches patient to report any adverse reactions immediately			
22. Assembles equipment prior to attempting venipuncture			
23. Washes hands			
24. Selects appropriate site for venipuncture			
25. Applies tourniquet properly			
26. Preps the venipuncture site according to institutional policy without subsequent contamination			
27. Successfully performs venipuncture with two (or fewer) attempts			
28. Removes the tourniquet			
29. Anchors needle with tape to prevent dislodgement			
30. Stabilizes venipuncture site			
31. Checks for patency of vein by instilling 5–7 cc of normal saline			
32. Reconfirms vein patency periodically by obtaining blood backflow either by aspirating or occluding flow of solution			
33. Flushes tubing upon completion of one drug before administering another drug			
34. Injects drugs at the appropriate speed to prevent untoward sensations/complications			
35. Takes appropriate action should infiltration of a drug occur			
36. Observes for allergic or hypersensitivity reactions to the drugs and takes appropriate action should either occur			
37. If using a venous access device, demonstrates skill in usage and maintenance of the device			
38. Flushes IV tubing with a sufficient amount of saline to clear the line prior to removing the needle			
39. Removes the needle, elevates the extremity, and instructs the patient to apply pressure to the site			
40. Applies a dressing to the venipuncture site			
41. Instructs patient on post-treatment care and precautions			
42. Disposes of equipment in proper container according to institutional policies and procedures			
43. Documents procedure in the medical record according to institutional policies and procedures			

APPENDICES

Appendix 6. Clinical Practicum Evaluation: Part II

The nurse performs the following activities at a satisfactory level. If there has not been an opportunity to carry out a particular activity, indicate N/A (not applicable) in the space provided. Under comments, give examples of how the nurse met each objective or performed each activity.

	Yes	No
1. Participates in interdisciplinary care planning with physicians and other healthcare professionals (e.g., home care, dietary) Comments:		
2. Anticipates complications of chemotherapy and takes action to prevent/minimize the complications Comments:		
3. Involves patient and family in care planning, and attempts to establish interventions specific to the individual needs of the patient Comments:		
4. Instructs patient on hair/scalp care and measures to minimize hair loss and preserve body image Comments:		
5. Reviews laboratory indices and appropriately instructs a myelosuppressed patient regarding conservation of energy, infection, and bleeding precautions Comments:		
6. Identifies patients at risk for stomatitis and instructs the patient on oral hygiene and preventive measures Comments:		
7. Demonstrates knowledge of the use of drug therapy, relaxation, and diversional therapies in the prevention and management of nausea and vomiting Comments:		
8. Instructs patient regarding the prevention and management of gastrointestinal complications (e.g., constipation, diarrhea) Comments:		
9. Identifies and takes nursing action in the prevention or management of a potential/actual allergic reaction Comments:		
10. Takes appropriate precautions in the preparation, handling, and disposal of chemotherapy Comments:		
11. Demonstrates knowledge and skill in assessment, management, and follow-up care of extravasation Comments:		
12. Demonstrates skill in assessing the patient's need for a venous access device and the factors to be considered in selecting one type of device over another for a particular patient Comments:		
13. Demonstrates knowledge of research trials through participation in data collection, drug administration, patient education, and follow-up Comments:		

Progression of Intravenous Extravasation

Photos courtesy of the Cleveland Clinic Foundation, Shirley M. Gullo, RN, MSN, OCN®

Photo 1.
Erythema and blistering

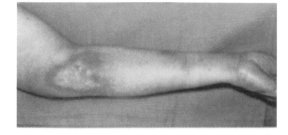

Photo 2.
Painful erythema and
beginning tissue necrosis

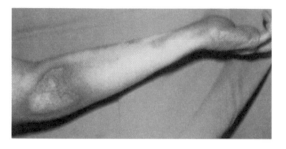

Photo 3.
Progressive necrosis and
ulceration

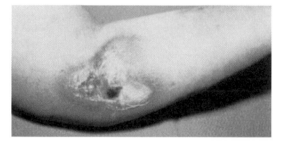

Photo 4.
Surrounding tissue begin-
ning to heal

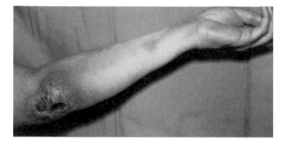

Photo 5.
Healing tissue with resulting
tissue defect

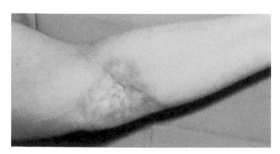
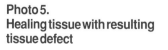

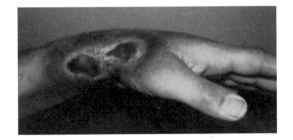

Photo 6.
Severe tissue necrosis second-ary to vesicant extravasation

Photo courtesy of Rita Wickham, MS, RN, OCN®

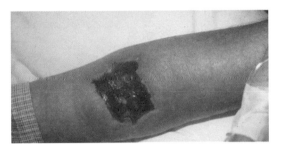

Photo 7.
Antecubital fossa extravasation

Index

INDEX